The Master Cleanse

Coach

Expert Coaching for You and Your Friends

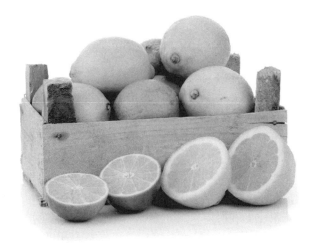

Peter Glickman

Author of the best-selling
Master Cleanse book,
*Lose Weight, Have More Energy
& Be Happier in 10 Days*

The Master Cleanse Coach:
Expert Coaching for Yourself and Others

© 2013 by Peter Glickman, Inc.
Published by Peter Glickman, Inc.
Clearwater, Florida
www.themastercleanse.com

Editing, design and layout by
Maggy Graham, www.wordsandpicturespress.com

Also by Peter Glickman:
  Lose Weight, Have More Energy & Be Happier in 10 Days
  The Lemonade Diet: A Master Cleanse Audio CD
  Anti-Aging, Detoxification & Weight Loss (DVD)
  Master Cleanse Coach, iPhone App
  Master Cleanse Coach, Android App

Printed in the United States of America.

Federal guidelines for testimonials require that typical results must be clearly stated. Typical Master Cleanse results are weight loss. (Ten days on a 660–1320 calorie per day diet will do that for people.)

Also, results vary (as though you haven't already seen that for yourself). So, you may not gain an improved mental outlook, healthier looking skin, more energy, clearer thinking; or the relief, temporary or permanent, of: asthma, arthritis pain, high blood pressure, skin rashes, digestive problems, etc. that are sometimes mentioned, but are not typical for everyone who does the Master Cleanse.

THE INFORMATION GIVEN IN THIS BOOK IS SOLELY FOR EDUCATIONAL PURPOSES. IT IS NOT INTENDED AS MEDICAL ADVICE. ANYONE WHO FOLLOWS IT DOES SO VOLUNTARILY.

Dedication

"In nothing do men approach so nearly to the Gods, as in giving health to men." Cicero

THIS BOOK IS DEDICATED TO EVERYONE WHO WANTS TO HELP OTHERS.

It is also dedicated to those who have the ability to observe for themselves rather than to listen to authorities who learned by memorizing prior authorities who never observed for themselves.

William Harvey, the doctor who first observed and then announced that the heart—not the lungs—circulated the blood, well understood that problem. He wrote (translated from 17th century English):

> I tremble to speak the truth of what I have discovered because it may make all mankind my enemies. Habit and popular opinion become second nature. Old ideas once planted, sprout deep roots and respect for our elders influences all men. Still, the die is cast and I must follow my love of truth and trust in the honesty of civilized minds.
>
> …
>
> Those who seek truth and knowledge, never consider themselves so thoroughly educated that they are not interested in learning more from anyone they can. They are not so narrow-minded to believe that the science taught them by their elders is so complete that there is nothing left to learn. On the contrary, many maintain we still don't know everything. True scientists do not so completely accept all they've been told that they cease to believe their own senses and deny and desert their friend, the Truth.

(*The Motion of the Heart and Blood*, William Harvey, 1628)

Fasting in general and juice fasting in particular have fallen out of favor in the last hundred years. A hundred years ago it was common to hear doctors and ministers encourage people to fast to regain and maintain vibrant good health as well as find themselves closer to the Holy Spirit. Yet there are some bright lights still among us.

Alan Cott, MD, wrote a bestselling book in 1975 called *Fasting: The Ultimate Diet*. He followed it with *Fasting as a Way of Life* a year later. In that later book (pp. 68-69), he said:

> "If fasting is so wondrous, the question might well be asked, Why aren't more of us in the medical profession championing it?"
>
> …
>
> "The primary discoveries of Harvey, Lister [washing hands to prevent spreading germs], Pasteur … and many others were vigorously resisted from within the profession. Rene Laennec was expelled from his medical society after inventing the stethoscope…"
>
> …
>
> "I find it incongruous that doctors inexperienced in the fast immediately talk about fasting in terms of danger, yet casually prescribe enormous doses of tranquilizers and sleeping pills for periods of many years, as well as antibiotics and other drugs having the potential for unpleasant, sometimes irreversible side effects, addiction, and a high incidence of [illness]."
>
> …
>
> "*The Journal of the American Medical Association* published the opinion that fasting provides the best method of self-discipline needed by the obese—'one that can be repeated with beneficial effect.'"

And most importantly, it is dedicated to Stanley Burroughs for developing the Master Cleanse and publishing it.

MAY YOU BRING VIBRANT GOOD HEALTH AND JOY TO YOURSELF AND OTHERS AND MAY YOUR LIFE BE BLESSED AS A RESULT.

Table of Contents

Table of Contents

Table of Contents

Introduction

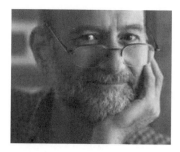

THE MASTER CLEANSE HAS ROUTINELY produced such remarkable results that it inspires others and therefore has survived without advertising. Surveys I conducted in 2005 and 2011 show the average person who completes a 10-day Master Cleanse inspires at least three more people to do the Master Cleanse.

This second book was written to accomplish two purposes: answer your questions and those of your friends. Most likely, they will ask you how to do it and call you with questions once they begin. I hope this book helps you get them the best possible results. After all, they are your friends.

Do not worry if you have only done one 10-day or longer Master Cleanse. After I did my first Master Cleanse, I had many people asking me questions. I just opened *The Master Cleanser*, found the answer and read it to them on the phone. This task is now much easier with this book or my other book, *Lose Weight, Have More Energy & Be Happier in 10 Days*. They both have the most frequent questions broken out alphabetically and a table of contents. The Master Cleanser has neither of those.

If You Want It Done Right ...

You have heard it said, "If you want it done right, do it yourself." This is especially true when it comes to your health. Your body is different from other bodies in blood type, capacity to handle work, food, sugar, alcohol, etc. Penicillin will kill the bacteria causing your infection, but if you are allergic to it you could die instead. So, you must learn what works for you and your body. You, factually, are the only person who can make the determination of what is helpful or not for you. Health professionals can give you valuable information and do other things, but ultimately, the buck stops with you. So you have to learn to use good judgment along with your experience and that includes determining if the information in this book is useful to you.

The information in this book is solely for your education. It is not intended as medical advice or to diagnose, treat, cure or prescribe. It is for you to decide whether to follow it. If you do, it must be because you have determined that it would be good for you to try it.

Best wishes for your vibrant good health,

Peter Glickman

Part I
Key Coaching Points

COACHING YOUR FRIENDS ON THE MASTER CLEANSE IS USUALLY JUST as easy as doing it yourself *if* you know the key points and have the right tools. These are:

I.   What you need to know as a coach: Part I of this book.

II. What you and your friends need to know to do the Master Cleanse: Parts II and III of this book or my book, *Lose Weight, Have More Energy & Be Happier in 10 Days*. Available as a paperback or digital download from www.TheMasterCleanse.com/store.

III. Scientific support so you have some ammunition for those who reject the Master Cleanse without any real knowledge or experience with it. This support can be found in the third edition of *Lose Weight, Have More Energy & Be Happier in 10 Days* in the "Perspective" and "Anti-Aging" chapters.

IV. The "bible" of the Master Cleanse is of course *The Master Cleanser* by Stanley Burroughs, the original developer of the Master Cleanse. (Available as a paperback from www.TheMasterCleanse.com/store.) The only thing I have done differently is to recommend taking probiotics after one returns to solid food. So, it is not really any change to Burroughs' remarkable work.

V.   *The Master Cleanse Journal* for your friends. (Available as a digital download only from www.TheMasterCleanse.com/store.) This has all the actions necessary for the cleanse; places for before and after pictures and comments for four 10-day cleanses, two 20-day cleanses or one 40-day cleanse; and some helpful and inspirational quotations.

VI. A legal release form in the back of this book in case you decide to coach the Master Cleanse for money and are not a licensed health care practitioner. (*Be sure to check this with your attorney as I am not an attorney and local laws differ.*) This would be done on the basis that a person wishing on their own to do the Master Cleanse has asked you as a Master Cleanse enthusiast to coach them, just as a runner might pay a running coach. *You must not prescribe or treat them for any illness nor diagnose them with any illness unless you are a licensed health care practitioner.* However, many people are enthusiastic about doing the Master Cleanse for weight loss, detoxification or health maintenance. They certainly have a right to ask someone who knows more about it to coach them. Have people sign this *before* you coach them.

To ensure you do not miss important points, I have marked them with an exclamation mark, like the one at the beginning of this paragraph.

1. What You Need To Know To Do A Good Job

As a coach, these are the things you need to know to do a good job:

1. What you should and should not say

2. Who should do the Master Cleanse and who should not?

3. For best results, do not change the Master Cleanse. Only promote it as developed by Stanley Burroughs.

4. What are detoxification and detox symptoms?

5. What is or is not a detox symptom?

6. Should you encourage someone to continue or quit?

7. Why does the Master Cleanse work?

8. Where can you find good answers to the most common questions?

9. Coaching tips

2. What you should and should not say

The first thing to know about the Master Cleanse is never tell someone they should do the cleanse. I know that may shock you, but it is true and I actually never do it. "Wait," you say, "You have written a book about it. You have a website devoted to it. You do interviews and newsletters." Yes, that is all true, but nowhere do I say a particular person should do the cleanse. I am very enthusiastic on what it has done for me and I frequently promote others' benefits, but *I never tell a particular person they should do the cleanse.*

There are two reasons for this. The first is that in the United States, it is illegal to diagnose, prescribe, treat or cure a disease unless you are a licensed health practitioner. The second reason is much more important. The Master Cleanse has a built-in protection mechanism. People who are too toxic to do the cleanse will not even try to go without eating for a few days. So, please, talk all you want about the wonders and benefits of the cleanse, but when it comes to a particular person, let them decide whether they want to try it or not.

Please be aware that I am not a lawyer and am not familiar with the laws of the more than 100 countries to which I have shipped Master Cleanse books and supplies from my web store (www.TheMasterCleanse.com/store/). So, you need to verify that the advice I have given in this book follows your local laws.

You need to know there are people whose bodies have too many toxins and should not do the Master Cleanse. I will tell you which ones a little later, but there are two more things you should never do. First, never tell someone what's wrong with them: "Oh, you've got Candida." In most countries, once again, if you are not licensed, you cannot diagnose diseases.

The other thing you should not do is tell someone that something will happen for them in particular. Here are examples of questions where you have to be careful with your reply: "Peter, can I lose 15 pounds in 15 days?" "Will these terrible headaches be gone tomorrow?" "Are these ------------------ detox symptoms or should I see a doctor?" These questions lead into the dangerous territory of diagnosing, prescribing, treating and curing. You are a coach, not a licensed health care practitioner. You want to educate, not diagnose or treat. So, the best answers for these questions are:

- "Many people lose a pound a day: however, everybody is unique."

- "Most caffeine headaches occur only in the beginning and disappear after 1–4 days, usually in 2 or less."

- "That is a very common detox symptom." (If it is. More about what is and isn't later)

- "Most detox symptoms disappear or lessen with the next morning's eliminations. Let's see how it is tomorrow."

Keep in mind, if someone wants to see a licensed health care practitioner, never talk them out of it.

You will notice I never use the term "doctor," although most people use it. I use the term "licensed health care practitioner" to remind people that there are many kinds of licensed healers who use cheaper and more beneficial means of healing people in the long run. Broken bones and accidents are the exception.

Never tell anyone to stop taking or reduce medication *prescribed* by a licensed health care practitioner, unless you are one yourself. People on the Master Cleanse *should* stop taking any vitamins, supplements or over-the-counter drugs, but this does not mean anything that is *prescribed*. If they decide to stop taking or reduce medications on their own, that is their right, but unless you are licensed you cannot and should not tell them to do that. It is illegal in the US.

If they feel their current licensed health care practitioner will not be cooperative, you can *suggest* they see another licensed health care practitioner for a second opinion. Again, remind them that licensed "health care practitioner" could be a chiropractor, traditional Chinese medical doctor, naturopath (doctor who uses natural methods to permit the body to heal itself) or others.

2. Who should and who should not do the Master Cleanse?

Anyone who has undergone chemotherapy within the last 6 months should not do the Master Cleanse. It detoxifies too fast. Max Gerson, MD, who began researching the nutritional basis of cancer in 1948 and had many successful "cures" (remissions for more than 5 years), used a detoxification method as part of his treatment. He found that a portion of each chemotherapy dose stayed in the body and was released during detoxification. Releasing these residual doses could be very serious.

Anyone who is healing from a major wound or major surgery should not do the Master Cleanse until they are completely healed. The

Master Cleanse has no protein. This is not a problem for a month or more according to several licensed health care practitioners who fasted patients extensively in their practices: Herbert Shelton, ND, Joel Fuhrman, MD, Alan Cott, MD, Yuri Nikolayev, MD, and Otto Buchinger, MD. However for people who need to rebuild tissue, healing should be complete before doing the Master Cleanse or any fast.

Patients on blood thinning medications who do the Master Cleanse should liaise with their prescribing licensed health care practitioner because cayenne pepper is known to be a very effective natural blood thinner. Therefore, to avoid over-thinning the blood, the dosage of the medication may very well need to be reduced.

Likewise, patients on medication to reduce high blood pressure should liaise with their prescribing licensed health care practitioner because fasting has been shown by scientific studies to reduce high blood pressure. So, to avoid a severe drop in blood pressure, the dosage of the medication will likely need to be reduced. ("Medically supervised water-only fasting in the treatment of hypertension," *Journal of Manipulative Physiological Therapeutics*, 2001 & "Medically supervised water-only fasting in the treatment of borderline hypertension," *Journal of Alternative and Complementary Medicine*, 2002)

Patients who are on strong psychiatric drugs should discontinue their medications in conjunction with a licensed health care practitioner or should check out the program at www.TheRoadBack.org before doing the Master Cleanse. Many of these drugs have serious side effects when a person tries to come off them "cold turkey."

At one time, I said pregnant or nursing women should not do the Master Cleanse. This was based on the idea that it might be possible for toxins the mother is eliminating to enter the embryo or fetus. In seven years, I have not heard of a single case of this. In fact, I received an email from a midwife who wrote that in her 30-year practice she has had a number of mothers use the Master Cleanse with no ill effect. However, I recommend better safe than sorry.

Children in their rapidly growing years need protein and therefore should be discouraged from doing the Master Cleanse for 10 days or more. However, if they are not feeling well and have no desire for food, they should be permitted to drink only lemonade until they desire more substantial food. This is not to be taken as prescribing

! the Master Cleanse for children who are ill, but rather permitting children's bodies to heal themselves.

● People who are allergic to "everything" or those who are more than 60 pounds overweight *may* be too toxic to do the Master Cleanse. You do not have to prohibit them from doing it because they will quit the cleanse if it becomes too much. However, they should follow the instructions on page 65, "Severe detox symptoms," if their detox symptoms get to be too uncomfortable.

If someone is truly allergic to citrus, there is no way to do the Master Cleanse.

3. For best results, do not change the Master Cleanse. Only promote it as developed by Stanley Burroughs. Beware of alterations!

That title says it all, but I want to emphasize it to make the point.

The Master Cleanse made its way from 1976, when Stanley Burroughs published *The Master Cleanser* and *Healing For The Age Of Enlightenment*, to the present by delivering great results as a detox diet. In 2006 with my book, Robin Quivers (Howard Stern's producer), Beyonce and *The New York Times*, the Master Cleanse was suddenly a very popular weight loss diet. In 2003 when I put Master Cleanse information on my website, there were perhaps 100 web pages on it. By 2010, there were 1 ½ million! In the same time, the number of media shows and articles went from nearly zero to hundreds.

Unfortunately many of those shows, articles and web pages were written by people who wanted attention and advertising, but were not very careful with their facts. In 2006, *The New York Daily News* published a story by Jane Ridley in August 2006 saying each lemonade drink contained 32 oz. of water! Even when I brought the mistake up to the writer and the editor, they never corrected it.

In February 2009, *Us Weekly* ran a story saying the Master Cleanse included eating fish and quoting an "expert" saying he would do two days on and one day off for up to seven days. The Master Cleanse is a minimum of 10 days. Advising less immediately brands the speaker as one who doesn't know very much about the Master Cleanse and certainly has never done it. The advice to do two days on and one day off is even worse advice because days two and three are the worst days repeated over and over! Print media is not the only area of misinformation. One of the more popular Master Cleanse eBooks on the Internet, *Master Cleanse Secrets*, has an incorrect recipe for the lemonade.

On the Internet, there have been three major alterations of the Master Cleanse. *Master Cleanse Secrets* by Raylin Sterling contains the wrong recipe for the lemonade and possibly suggests adding other things to the cleanse.

Mike Olaski on his website, www.TheMasterCleanse.org, wanted to be able to use the words "Lemonade Diet" as well as "Master Cleanse" to get more exposure on Google. So he created the concept of a 3-day "Ease in" before the Master Cleanse, so he could call the 10 days of lemonade the "Lemonade Diet". Thus he could write about the Master Cleanse and the Lemonade Diet and get more exposure. There is no ease in as part of the Master Cleanse. In fact, Stanley Burroughs, the developer, called it the Master Cleanse, the Master Cleanser, the Lemonade Diet and the Lemon Juice Diet. They are all names for the same thing.

Verbal instructions from one person to another are just as bad. I have been asked when do you drink the vegetable soup each day by someone who was told how to do it. Whether he misremembered on his own or whether the person telling him misremembered it makes no difference. He would not get great results with these altered instructions.

I bring these up to make the point that just like the children's game of telephone where one person whispers a message to another who whispers it to another, the Master Cleanse is what Stanley Burroughs developed and published. It will spread just as far as it produces great results and no further. So, even if you used grapefruit juice instead of orange juice to ease back to solid food and it worked for you, tell others to do it with orange juice just like Burroughs said. His directions have stood the test of time. **His instructions have consistently produced the best results for the most people for half a century!** And results are the name of the game!

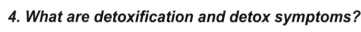

4. What are detoxification and detox symptoms?

Detoxification is the core of the Master Cleanse. You must understand it to understand what are and are not detox symptoms and what to do about them. This is the barrier to doing the Master Cleanse successfully and getting great results.

I have covered detoxification and its symptoms at length in "*Lose Weight, Have More Energy & Be Happier in 10 Days.*" Here, however, I will point out the *essentials* that will make you a good coach.

There are things that make you feel bad, tired and cause your body to function poorly. These are called toxins. They really exist.

You can get rid of these things.

Between the time these toxins are mobilized from where they are stored and when they are eliminated, they are capable of causing headaches, tiredness, irritability, cravings, boredom, wanting to quit the cleanse, rashes, colds, etc. They do not *always* do this.

When they do cause detox symptoms, the symptoms generally reduce or disappear within three days, usually with the next morning's eliminations. They rarely, if ever, last the entire cleanse.

If people know two things about detox symptoms, they can complete the full ten days of the Master Cleanse successfully. 1) Detox symptoms are milestones that indicate improvement is occurring. 2) These symptoms will usually not last more than a day or two.

It is the mistaken idea that they will have to live with these detox symptoms for the entire ten days that causes most people to quit and they usually quit on the most common days for detox symptoms: two, three, seven and fourteen.

Detox symptoms are avoided or minimized by doing evening laxative tea *every* night and the salt water flush or another cup of laxative tea *every* morning, which speed the toxins out of the body, hopefully before they create detox symptoms.

5. What is and is not a detox symptom?

This issue is only important when a friend wants to know whether to quit or continue. If someone has a detox symptom and it is not unbearable, they should continue.

It is unwise to quit on a day with a detox symptom. This is because the Master Cleanse will eliminate the toxins causing that detox symptom much faster than being on a normal diet. For example, a person may have turned on a rash that will go away in three days on the Master Cleanse, but may take more than a week to disappear on a normal diet.

However, if a friend actually has a problem that is not a detox symptom and it needs attention from a health care practitioner then that person should see a licensed health care practitioner.

While this list does not contain every detox symptom, it does contain the most common ones and some rules to help you identify most of the other detox symptoms:

a. Rashes and skin eruptions

b. Headaches on the first few days due to caffeine detoxification (This is an excellent proof that toxins really are eliminated on a detox diet.)

c. Burning eliminations (bowel movements)

d. Tiredness

e. Mental confusion

f. Irritability

g. Irregularity of a woman's period, whether spotting when it is not time, increased flow, reduced flow or missed periods

h. Aches or pains, particularly at the site of previous injuries or illnesses, such as hemorrhoids or broken bones

i. Hunger that does not go away with drinking more lemonade or water. This may occur if a person has taken diet pills in the past or a prescription medicine that has hunger or weight gain as a side effect.

j. Craving for a particular food, such as pizza or hamburgers

k. Dizziness

l. Nausea

m. Boredom or wanting to quit the cleanse

n. Cold-like symptoms, runny nose, etc.

o. Coated/furry tongue

p.   Trouble sleeping, usually only during the first few nights

q.   Unusual or especially vivid dreams

r.   Detox symptoms are *very* common on days 2, 3, 7, 14, 21, etc. These days may be off by one, for example day one or day four may have detox symptoms.

6. Should you encourage someone to continue or quit?

● You must always make it clear to your friends that the decision to continue or quit is *always* theirs. You are only providing them with others' experiences so they can make up their mind.

● The reason for this is two-fold. Legally, you cannot diagnose, prescribe, treat or cure, which you would be doing if you instructed someone to continue. You would be diagnosing they had a detox symptom and prescribing they continue the cleanse.

● Much more important than that however, the Master Cleanse is self-protective and must be kept that way. A person cleansing will quit before they get into a serious problem.

● So, when a friend says, "I feel terrible and have this awful rash. I think I want to quit." First let them know you heard them and can relate to what they said. Then, find out on which day they are, for example, day two or seven. If it is within one day of a common detox day, be sure to remind them of that fact.

● Then, tell them, "Detox days, when a person on the cleanse feels bad for a day or two, are very common. Rashes are also common. Most detox symptoms reduce or go away within three days." Wait and get their response to the information you just gave them. If they still want to quit and you are confident it is a detox symptom, you can tell them of your own detox symptom experiences or someone else's.

● If your friend still wants to quit, let them. Never make him/her wrong for quitting. Cleansing is an ongoing process, not a one-time event where you get a report card and never have another chance. You want them to feel they can talk to you and tell you anything without you making them wrong or condemning them.

Let them know that they can always try again later or use a slower method of detoxification (page 45) and then try the Master Cleanse again.

7. Why does the Master Cleanse work?

a. Fasting

! Fasting is one of the, if not *the*, most powerful natural methods of rejuvenating body and mind and was used before written history. It is naturally followed by animals, which refuse to eat when sick. It permits the body to redirect the energy the body normally uses for digestion and elimination (30% of its total energy) to detoxification and rejuvenation.

! Nearly every major religion includes fasting. Hippocrates, the Father of Western Medicine, used fasting to allow the body to heal itself.

It is important to understand the relationship between fasting and health, so you will know that consuming *anything* solid will reduce the effectiveness of the Master Cleanse. Likewise, consuming *anything* other than the lemonade for nourishment will reduce the effectiveness of the fast. This includes chewing gum as chewing stimulates saliva and production of stomach acid in preparation for digestion. This robs the body of energy to rebuild. Chewing gum also requires sweeteners, which are either artificial or sugar. Neither is beneficial.

Papers presented at the 2000 Buryatia, Russia Medical Conference on Fasting show it is effective for obesity, general health, gout, high blood pressure, cardiovascular disease, ulcers, arthritis, nodules in internal organs, skin diseases, bacterial & viral infections in internal organs and mental problems such as psychoses, schizophrenia and neuroses.

Occasionally, a person eats a bite of something on the Master Cleanse and still gets results. Then they tell others it is okay to eat. I cannot say this enough: The largest number of people will get the best results if they follow Stanley Burroughs' instructions *exactly*. You need to know that fasting is a great deal of the power of the Master Cleanse so you will not waiver in your advice.

b. Detoxification

I have covered this above and in *Lose Weight, Have More Energy & Be Happier in 10 Days*. Detoxification is the core of the Master Cleanse.

c. Calorie Restriction

A 30% calorie restricted diet, which still provides optimum nutrition, is the *only* method of life extension that has been proven in scientific studies. It also reduces age-related diseases, such as heart disease, cancer, diabetes and obesity as shown in scientific studies. (See the chapter on Anti-Aging in *Lose Weight, Have More Energy & Be Happier in 10 Days*.)

d. Rehydrating the body

In *Your Body's Many Cries for Water*, the author, an MD, makes the case that chronic dehydration is the root cause of most physical diseases and explains the damaging effects of dehydration. He discusses the role of water in the body and his belief that water can restore and maintain your health.

Emphasizing his point, dehydration is the main reason for hospital admissions of more than 25% of long-term nursing home residents according to a 2004 study printed in *Gerontology*. That study and others found that more than half of all hospital patients with dehydration die if not adequately treated. So, you can see it is vital to drink the minimum 6 lemonades a day.

8. Where can you find good answers to the most common questions?

Did you notice I said "good answers," not just "answers"? This is because there is a lot of incorrect information about the Master Cleanse on the Internet and even in magazines and newspapers. Remember the examples I gave above? (See "For best results, do not change the Master Cleanse. Only promote it as developed by Stanley Burroughs" above, if you forgot.)

Many people are enthusiastic about their Master Cleanse experience and want to share it. Sometimes what they say will echo your own experiences. Sometimes it is fun to read or hear of others' experiences, but *when it comes to coaching stick with Burroughs.* He developed it.

9. Coaching Tips

● Attitude is very important. If you have a generous, caring, supportive attitude, your friends will carry that away and mirror it to others; whether they do the cleanse or not; whether they succeed or not. But, if you are commanding and refuse to listen to them, they will carry that away as well.

● Mental and spiritual certainty is vital to health. Let your friends' certainty come from their own observations and decisions. Help them base those decisions on their experiences and conclusions after hearing of others' experiences from you—either those you know of directly or from reading *Lose Weight, Have More Energy & Be Happier in 10 Days.*

● Information and decisions forced on someone are at best short-term solutions. Truth arrived at from personal inspection and experience forms a solid foundation for a better life. So, always educate and encourage; never command or order.

● Do not argue with anyone. Listen to what they have to say. Let them know you heard what they said. State what you know to be true. Repeat. If they have not seen the wisdom of your point after two or three tries, leave it alone. You cannot force someone to do what you believe is right. If you follow this advice you will not get into useless arguments that leave both parties upset. Who knows? They may see the wisdom of your point after they try it their way.

● If someone wants to alter the Master Cleanse from Stanley Burroughs' directions all you can do is offer the advice that it has been tested for more than half a century and works. The greatest number of people will get the most benefits by doing it his way. Request they pass on Burroughs' instructions whether they decide to follow them personally or not. Do not get into an argument. See the paragraph above.

● When you are trying to discover why a friend is having trouble and you can see nothing unusual, ask them to tell you exactly what they do each day. Exactly how do they mix the salt water or lemonade? Do not let them say, "I follow the recipe." Make them tell you how much of each ingredient they use, where they get their lemon juice, etc. I have discovered people using the wrong recipe or bottled juice, but only after pressing them for the exact specifics. Up until that time, they said, "I followed the directions" or "I used the recipe to mix the lemonade."

- If, after you have explained something, you suspect your friend still doesn't know exactly what to do, ask them to tell you in detail what they are going to do on that point. Then you can see if they have it correct. Some people need repetition. This technique will allow you to discover which people need it and which don't.

For more information on coaching the Master Cleanse, join the "Members Only" section at www.TheMasterCleanse.com and may this information bring you as many grateful thank you's as it has me.

And if you are interested in becoming a certified Master Cleanse Coach, please email info@MasterCleanseCoach.com.

Please note: I am not an attorney and even if I were, I am not familiar with the laws of every state. Therefore the General Release and Waiver on the last page of this book should be reviewed by an attorney licensed to practice in the state in which you live.

Part II
How to Do the Master Cleanse

● Shopping List

IMPORTANT NOTE: These quantities are based on six glasses of lemonade per day for the minimum of ten days. You should drink six to twelve glasses of lemonade per day. So, you may have to multiply these quantities if you drink more glasses per day or go longer than ten days.

- Books: *Lose Weight, Have More Energy & Be Happier in 10 Days* by Peter Glickman and/or *The Master Cleanser* by Stanley Burroughs

- 30 large lemons, 60 limes or small lemons, or a combination. Only buy half this amount and the other half later, if you buy organic, which is preferred. Organic spoils faster than conventional fruit.

- 64 fluid ounces organic Grade B maple syrup or the darkest organic maple syrup you can find

- At least four ounces of sea salt that does not say "iodized" or "iodine added"

- At least six teaspoons (about one half ounce) of cayenne pepper powder, not capsules. Regular cayenne is about 30,000 heat units. You can use hotter if you like.

- A box of at least ten herbal laxative tea bags. I recommend those teas with 50 percent senna rather than pure senna leaf tea.

- At least eight gallons of spring, purified or distilled water without added fluoride or chlorine for the lemonade, salt water flush and a cup of laxative tea each evening. Fluoride was used for decades as rat poison. It is very injurious to human health and studies have shown it to increase the risk of cancer and hip fractures.

- One box or bottle of probiotics to be taken per the directions on the bottle or box after you return to eating solid food.

- These ingredients should be easy to find at any health food store, not grocery store. If you cannot find these easily, you can order them at www.TheMasterCleanse.com/store, or if you have Peter Glickman's Master Cleanse Coach app for Android or iPhone, use the "Books and Supplies" link.

- Do not buy cayenne in capsules. According to Dr. Richard Schulze, a master herbalist, people who take cayenne capsules do not receive much of the benefit of the cayenne. The nerve endings in the mouth respond almost instantly to send blood throughout the body. This whole process is missed if you take capsules. People who "hate" it or "can't stand it" have simply used too much for their first taste. It is a learned taste. The way to handle "hating" it is to start by adding only a sprinkle and then gradually build up the amount as you can tolerate it.

- Do not buy pre-mixed powders or bottled juice. They must be pasteurized by law, which kills most of the enzymes in the lemon/lime juice. I know from the personal experience of coaching someone who was using bottled lemon juice that it did not produce very good results until she switched to fresh squeezed lemon juice. Likewise, avoid all powders and pills for the same reason: dehydrated powders do not have the same effectiveness as fresh enzymes.

- Do not buy additional vitamins or supplements. Burroughs says three times in his book, *The Master Cleanser*, not to take any other supplements. Fasting has been a powerful and natural way to heal and rejuvenate the body for thousands of years. Animals instinctively fast when they are ill. The

Master Cleanse is a juice fast. Adding anything to it merely reduces the power of the fast.

- Do not buy kits that contain less than 64 ounces of organic maple syrup. Some providers try to lower their price by shorting the amount of maple syrup because maple syrup is the most expensive item in the cleanse.

Quick Start

They say you cannot please everyone, but I am going to try. There are those people who like to have all the information before they start. I understand you because I am like that most of the time. However, sometimes I just want to jump in and start. If I need the details, I will get them when I need them. For you, I have created this Quick Start. Just begin here and consult the alphabetical table of contents for whatever details you need when you need them.

Read the Shopping List before this section, if you have not already done so.

- The night before and every night of the cleanse, drink one cup of herbal laxative tea before bed.

- Before drinking any lemonade, each day of the cleanse, drink thirty-two ounces of spring, purified or distilled water with two TEASPOONS of sea salt.

- During each day of the cleanse, drink 6 to 12 glasses of lemonade:

    > 2 tablespoons (1 fluid ounce) of fresh-squeezed lemon/lime juice

    > 2 tablespoons (1 fluid ounce) of organic, Grade B maple syrup

    > 1/10 teaspoon of cayenne pepper or to taste

    > 8 ounce of medium-hot (or cold if you prefer) spring, purified or distilled water.

- As much herbal mint tea and/or water as you wish.

- Do not eat anything else; no solid food. The only exception is prescribed medications. Do not discontinue prescriptions without consulting a licensed health care practitioner.

- Breaking the cleanse:

  First day after the cleanse, slowly drink several glasses of freshly squeezed orange juice. If you experience any digestive problems, dilute the orange juice with water.

  Second day, freshly squeezed orange juice all day for vegetarians. Others should make a homemade vegetable soup in the afternoon from several different vegetables, such as carrots, celery, potatoes, onions, tomatoes, green peppers, zucchini, beans, peas, lentils, brown rice, and dehydrated veggies or spices. Use sea salt sparingly. No meat or meat stock. Drink mostly the broth for dinner.

  Third day, freshly squeezed orange juice in the morning for vegetarians, followed by fresh fruit for lunch and a fruit or raw vegetable salad for dinner. Others drink orange juice in the morning, have the rest of the soup for lunch and eat a vegetarian dinner limited to fruit, salad or vegetables.

- I recommend on the third day after the cleanse, you begin to take probiotics per the instructions on the box or bottle to replace any good bacteria that may have been flushed out of you.

More Details

1. Length of Time, and Frequency

The Master Cleanse should be done for at least ten days. Burroughs says it can be done for forty or more days. I've personally done it more than nineteen times from ten to twenty-eight days (and once for three days). Burroughs is right about ten days being the minimum. The three-day Master Cleanse left me feeling as though nothing had been accomplished. I can hear you saying, "Ten days?! Is he crazy?" Amazingly, you will not be hungry and you will have more energy than you felt before the Master Cleanse.

In addition to my own longer Master Cleanses, I know of three other people who have done it for twenty days. All of us found that there were spiritual gains after eight or ten days: a clarity of purpose, a sense of focus, a feeling of well being, and a discovery that our natural emotion is one of cheerful satisfaction.

Burroughs says the best sign that the Master Cleanse is complete is a clear, pink tongue. Your tongue will definitely get coated and turn white and possibly other colors. Not everyone continues until their tongue is clear and pink. If you want to quit sooner, you can. The Master Cleanse is not like a school grade that you only do once. You can do it three or four times a year, each time detoxing more. Most stop at ten days regardless of tongue color. However, ten days is long enough to make a major change in your weight, health and mental outlook.

How soon can you do another Master Cleanse? It's best to space out your Master Cleanses by three or four months and eat lots of fresh greens and salads in between or drink daily green smoothies. You need to build up your calcium, magnesium and potassium reserves because the body uses those alkaline minerals to neutralize the toxins before they are eliminated. Very rarely (three out of a thousand), a person has done a Master Cleanse every month for several months in a row, which resulted in temporary hair loss. It was handled by taking lots of vitamins and minerals, but it is better to avoid that.

Refined sugar reduces calcium in the bones and teeth as the body needs to balance the blood chemistry after eating sugar, and it uses calcium to do that, which it will pull from the teeth and bones if there is no alkaline mineral reserve. Perhaps the epidemic of osteoporosis is no more than the popularity of a diet with too much sugar and not enough fresh, raw greens! By the way, milk is not a good source of calcium for building reserves. It is too hard for most people to digest it.

2. Laxative Tea

Drink one cup of herbal laxative tea before bed on the night before and every night thereafter while you are on the cleanse, unless you have diarrhea. (Diarrhea is NOT watery eliminations within two hours of drinking the salt water flush.) If you have diarrhea, discontinue the laxative tea and salt water flush until it stops. You can buy herbal laxative tea in most health food stores. There are two types I am aware of: pure senna tea and combinations of senna with other herbs. I recommend herbal laxative bags with 50 percent senna leaf rather than pure senna leaf tea. Senna is a powerful laxative and too much may cause cramps, particularly in the later days of a cleanse when there is little in the intestines. Although not painful, they are uncomfortable and can cause unnecessary concern. If such cramps do occur, they can be turned off quite quickly by drinking water or lemonade.

I personally did not have any problem with senna until my third Master Cleanse. Then I felt uncomfortably strong contractions and switched to a combination tea. Occasionally, when I run out of the combination, I'll make half a cup and dilute it.

I have been asked (rarely) if senna is addictive or will cause damage. I have never seen or heard of damage or addiction with any of the thousands of people who have done the Master Cleanse of whom I am aware. Perhaps 10 percent have reported uncomfortable cramps. In my experience, the cramps have disappeared when the salt water or lemonade is drunk and can be avoided by using the combination teas. The senna box warns not to give it to children or to drink more than two cups per day. The combination box says not to drink more than four cups per day and half that for children from six to twelve years old.

3. Salt Water Flush

Before drinking any lemonade, each day of the cleanse, drink a quart of water with two teaspoons of non-iodized sea salt. Drink it all at once or as close to that as you can. Non-iodized sea salt is sea salt that does not say "Iodine added" or "Iodized." It is easier to drink than bleached pure white table salt. The other reason to use non-iodized sea salt is that it contains vital trace minerals that your body needs. Non-iodized sea salt does not mean no iodine. It means no additional iodine has been added. Any brand will do. I personally recommend Light Grey Celtic Sea Salt, which can be found at most health food stores. Do not drink any lemonade or take any prescribed medications for a half hour after drinking the salt water.

This should produce several urgent and intense eliminations within an hour. If it does not, gradually increase the amount of sea salt. If that does not work, try a little less sea salt. These urgent eliminations generally take place for forty-five to sixty minutes. Plan two hours before you leave the house after drinking the salt water flush. After a couple days of salt water flushes, you can gauge how much time you need, but two hours is generally safe.

Some people have trouble with drinking the salt water. Be sure you stir the salt water so the salt is evenly distributed in the drink just before you drink it. It will be easier to drink and it is more effective. I believe it is very important to include it. So try everything you can. My wife found it helpful to drink it through a straw or to count the number of swallows as you drink it. Do not add anything to the salt water to make it taste better. Stay with the program. If you find that you absolutely cannot drink the salt water, Burroughs says you can drink another cup of herbal laxative tea in the morning instead. However, the laxative stimulates the muscles of the intestinal wall to contract and mechanically move the waste through. The salt water flushes whatever loose waste is in the digestive tract and the salt also helps to dissolve the mucus and waste.

- Many people have noticed that it is much easier to drink the salt water flush on later days of a cleanse. I believe this may be because the body reacts more dramatically when it has more mucus in the system and, as that gets cleaned out, the body has less reaction to the salt water flush.

The reason for two teaspoons of salt is to increase the weight (specific gravity) of the salt water until it matches the weight of blood. Specific gravity is how heavy the substance is compared to an equal volume of water. When the salt water and the blood are the same weight, the body will treat the salt water as though it were blood, not absorb the salt from the digestive system, and will just "flush" the salt water through the system instead of absorbing it.

- People who have recently been on the Atkins diet or any heavy meat and dairy diet may need two or three days before the flush produces eliminations. This is because meat and dairy are frequently hard to digest and build up waste that clogs the colon.

After the Master Cleanse, you may do the salt water flush whenever you want to clean your intestines. Just be sure to do it on an empty stomach.

4. The Drink: Lemons, Maple Syrup, Cayenne, Water

If you drink less than six glasses a day, you will not lose as much weight and may have more severe detox symptoms. Here are the recipes:

Ideal recipe, if freshly extracted sugar cane juice is available:

- 10 ounces of medium-hot or cold, freshly extracted sugar cane juice

- 2 tablespoons (1 fluid ounce) of fresh squeezed lemon/lime juice

- 1/10 teaspoon of cayenne pepper or to taste

- Next best recipe:

- 2 tablespoons (1 fluid ounce) of freshly squeezed lemon/lime juice

- 2 tablespoons (1 fluid ounce) of organic Grade B maple syrup

- 1/10 teaspoon of cayenne pepper or to taste

- 8 ounces of medium-hot (or cold if you prefer) spring, purified or distilled water

The enzymes in the lemon break down the layers of old waste in the colon. Although the lemon is acidic, it becomes alkaline when digested and the alkalinity helps neutralize the acidity of the toxic wastes. Try to get organic lemons from your local health food store, if possible, as they contain more minerals than non-organic ones. The lemon juice must be fresh squeezed, not bottled. The enzymes begin to break down within hours and heating (Pasteurizing) kills them completely. If you must prepare the drinks for most of the day—for taking to work, for example—prepare only that much and make fresh lemonade when you get home for the rest of the day. To make up more than one day's lemonade at one time or to try to save the squeezed lemon juice for another day will lose a great deal of the potency of the lemons.

Burroughs says to never to vary the amount of lemon juice in each drink. You can increase or decrease the maple syrup, but not the amount of the lemon juice.

The maple syrup supplies the sugar for energy and more importantly, it supplies the needed minerals. Use the darkest organic maple syrup you can find, which in the U.S. is Grade B. A is lighter than B. The darker the syrup, the more minerals. So try to get B if possible, but any organic grade will do. There is no Grade C anymore. If you are buying Canadian syrup, just get the darkest organic maple syrup you can find. The reason for organic is that some companies use formaldehyde in the process of tapping the trees. Organic grade B maple syrup can be found in most health food stores.

If you cannot find maple syrup, freshly extracted sugar cane juice makes the ideal lemonade drink. See the previous page for the recipe. A less-than-optimum substitute is sorghum, but Burroughs says it does not produce results as good. Use two tablespoons, the same amount as maple syrup.

If you are diabetic see the section "For Those With Diabetes or High Blood Pressure" below.

Agave nectar should not be used. Agave must be heated to make it sweet. The heating creates fructose and agave has more fructose than high fructose corn syrup, which was linked to obesity in a Princeton University study.[1]

Cayenne pepper contains Vitamin A, several B vitamins and Vitamin C and has been used by master herbalists for dilating blood vessels, dissolving mucus and feeding the heart. It is sold in several heat strengths as measured in heat units. If you do not usually eat hot food, buy the 30,000 heat unit cayenne. African Bird Pepper is 80,000 heat units. It is really hot.

---

1 "High-fructose corn syrup causes characteristics of obesity in rats: increased body weight, body fat and triglyceride levels," Bocarsly ME, Powell ES, Avena NM, Hoebel BG., *Pharmacology, biochemistry, and behavior*, Nov. 2010

I know I am repeating myself, but this is important. If you do not like cayenne pepper, you may be tempted to take capsules, leave it out or take a concentrated dose and then drink the lemonade without the pepper. Do not do these things. Cayenne acts like an accelerator pedal for the cleanse. It is a learned taste, meaning you have to try it a few times before you like it. So, if you do not like it, just add a tiny pinch to the first few drinks and gradually build up the amount as it is comfortable for you to do so.

Another reason not to take cayenne in capsules is the body must digest the capsule to gain the benefit of the cayenne. You are not eating anything that requires digestion to give your digestive system a chance to rest as well as cleanse itself. Since digestion uses 30 percent of the body's energy, you are gaining more usable energy by eliminating digestion. So, taking cayenne capsules should not be done.

5. Water/Mint Tea

In addition to the above, you may drink as much spring, distilled or purified water as you wish and occasionally some mint tea for a change. Do not use fluoridated water.

6. No Other Food or Drink

Nothing else is eaten or drunk on the Master Cleanse.

7. Breaking the Master Cleanse

Breaking the Master Cleanse diet correctly is very important! I have heard one second-hand story of someone coming off a long water fast, then going straight to overeating ribs and dessert, who then had serious medical problems. I do not know if this story is true, but I know personally that diving immediately back into a bad diet will make you feel very sick for a few hours. Correctly breaking the Master Cleanse is VERY important. I did it wrong once and had nausea and stomach pains for more than an hour. The longer your Master Cleanse is, the more important is how you break it.

I advise that you take one box or bottle of probiotics (following the directions on the bottle or box) after every cleanse to replace the good bacteria in your intestines that was eliminated on the cleanse. I discovered this after my third cleanse when I suddenly had intense cravings for "bad" food and taking probiotics eliminated the cravings for me. Probiotics make up 30 percent of the volume of your solid eliminations and so help to bring you back to regularity after the cleanse. They also produce vitamins A, B1, B2, B3, B12, and K; kill some of the disease-causing germs in your intestines; prevent bad bacteria (the bacteria that cause candida, for example) from getting out of control; and—some recent studies report—lower cholesterol and help in cases of irritable bowel syndrome (diarrhea, pain, and heightened food sensitivities). Antibiotics, while they are good for curing infections, destroy both good and bad bacteria. People, after taking antibiotics, should take probiotics to re-establish the good bacteria so necessary to health

If you usually eat meat, Burroughs says to break the fast slowly by drinking several glasses of orange juice for the first day and through the afternoon of the second. You may dilute the juice if you like or if you have any digestive problems. For dinner on the second day, drink mostly the broth of a homemade vegetable soup you make that afternoon from several different vegetables, beans and grains, such as carrots, celery, potatoes, onions, tomatoes, green peppers, zucchini, beans, peas, lentils, etc. No meat or meat stock. You may add brown rice and dehydrated veggies or spices, but use sea salt sparingly. The less you cook the soup, the better. You may have rye wafers with the soup, but not bread or crackers. Make enough for lunch the next day.

On the third day, drink orange juice in the morning. Have the rest of the soup for lunch. For dinner, eat whatever vegetarian salads, vegetables or fruit you wish. Begin eating your usual food the fourth day, although Burroughs recommends lemonade or fruit juice for breakfast on a continuing basis and a vegetarian diet as the best means of preserving life-long health.

If you are a vegetarian, drink fresh orange juice the first, second and morning of the third day. For lunch on the third day have raw fruit, with a raw fruit or vegetable salad for dinner. After that, eat normally.

If you have gas or digestive upset when breaking the fast, continue the Master Cleanse a few more days.

● For Those With Diabetes or High Blood Pressure

I have seen the Master Cleanse work very well for diabetics and I have heard of a case where it did not appear to work for a person. So, I am faithfully passing along Stanley Burroughs' instructions for diabetics as written in his book, *Healing for the Age of Enlightenment*. If you are a diabetic and wish to do the Master Cleanse, regularly test your blood sugar levels and do it in consulation with a licensed health care practitioner.

To start:

- 2 tablespoons (1 fluid ounce) of freshly squeezed lemon or lime juice

- Barely 1 tablespoon of molasses

- 1/10 teaspoon of cayenne pepper or to taste

- 8 ounces of medium-hot (or cold if you prefer) spring, purified or distilled water

- On following days, gradually increase the molasses by fractions of a tablespoon while monitoring blood sugar and reducing insulin. When 2 tablespoons of molasses have been achieved, check to see if it's possible to eliminate the insulin. Then use 2 tablespoons of maple syrup per drink.

You may drink as much herbal mint tea and/or water as you wish, providing that you drink at least six lemonades per day.

● If you are on medication for high blood pressure, be aware that the Master Cleanse lowers most people's blood pressure. It is well documented in scientific literature that fasting lowers blood pressure.[2] This means if you are on medication for high blood pressure you will need to coordinate with a licensed health care practitioner as it is extremely likely that your blood pressure will come down. Likewise, when standing up from a sitting or lying position, do so slowly as you may feel dizzy.

---

2 "Medically supervised water-only fasting in the treatment of hypertension," *Journal of Manipulative Physiological Therapeutics*, 2001

● If you are on anti-depression medication, consult with your prescribing health care practitioner. Some medications require food, others may require a lower dose while fasting. If you are interested in coming off these medications, visit If you cannot find these easily, you can order them at www.TheRoadBack.org. But do not combine their program with the Master Cleanse. Do their program, then the Master Cleanse.

● Detox Symptoms—the Good, the Bad and the Ugly

Detox symptoms are what you feel when toxins are mobilized, but not yet eliminated. Although detoxification symptoms are unpleasant, they ought to be desired. No one wants the feelings associated with detoxifying, but that is the purpose of the cleanse. If you are not detoxifying, you are not making progress and will not feel better afterward!

I place detox symptoms into five classes. Knowing these symptoms will be gone in a day or two, it is much easier to persevere and complete the cleanse.

1. Cravings. I have noticed I crave things for a few hours or a day. Usually after the next morning's elimination, the craving is gone and I feel better. As your body detoxifies (eliminates the toxic waste from) cooked meat, dairy products, etc., it craves the hamburger, pizza, ice cream, etc. that is being "peeled off" in layers. Paavo Airola discusses this concept on page 153 of his book *How to Get Well*. If you think about it, smokers who quit are immediately subject to intense cravings for the same toxins their bodies are eliminating now that they have been given the chance. The same thing is true of drug addicts.

     ● This is why Burroughs says addicts can more easily quit their habits while on the Master Cleanse. It helps reduce the cravings that are the largest barrier to quitting.

2. Tiredness. It should not be strange that toxins which age you and drain your energy should make you tired. When your body fights toxins, whether from detoxifying or from an infection, it diverts energy into healing and away from the energy you use to work and play. Toxins only make you tired until they are eliminated. That is why both the herbal

laxative tea and salt water flush are so important. They are the "Agitator" and "Rinse Cycle" of the Master Cleanse. Most people have a day or two when they feel tired. Give yourself permission to rest on those days.

3. Irritability, boredom, etc. The irritability of dieters is common knowledge. Among the reasons for this is that reduced eating allows the body to detoxify and one of the symptoms of detoxification is irritability. In this class of symptoms, I also include boredom, anxiety, wanting to "just chew something," and wanting to quit the Master Cleanse. It is quite remarkable how the next day's eliminations can change your attitude toward the Master Cleanse.

    When you get to Day 8 or so, you may discover for yourself that your natural mood is positive and cheerful. I have a friend in Georgia who told me how surprised he was that he was able to stay so upbeat during the Master Cleanse in the face of some serious problems.

4. Physical aches, pains, nausea, vomiting, etc. A few people on the Master Cleanse get headaches or other aches, in my experience perhaps 5 percent or less.

    Those who get headaches usually had a caffeine habit (coffee or soft drinks) before starting on the Master Cleanse. Detoxifying from caffeine with the Master Cleanse with the salt water flush and laxative tea is probably much easier than going off it "cold turkey." Caffeine headaches are usually one or two days. The longest I have heard was four days. Persist. Nausea and vomiting are much rarer, but not unheard of. Again these are detox symptoms and will go away.

    Other people may have aches and pains from previous illnesses for a few days before these aches and pains disappear a few days later. A friend had very severe hemorrhoids prior to the Master Cleanse. They appeared a few days after he started and went away a few days later. It was his impression that they would not be back.

5.   Hot or burning bowel movements. Toxins and other waste are acidic. I have found that when I eliminate old waste and other toxins, my bowel movements are actually hot. During my first Master Cleanse, my eliminations actually burned. I have also noticed that when I have serious detox symptoms as listed above, my eliminations the next morning are typically hot. This may be so bad in the first few days that you need to put some Vitamin E oil on your butt to soothe it. It acts within minutes.

Occasionally, someone will ask if it is the cayenne that burns. While cayenne in large quantities can temporarily cause hot bowel movements, this does not explain how—on a constant dose of cayenne—one can suddenly experience hot bowel movements after several days of normal temperatures. No, I am convinced it is the acidic toxins being eliminated.

In medicine, these detox symptoms are called Herxheimer Reactions. In alternative medicine, they are also called healing crises. They are a double-edged sword. Detox symptoms are a milestone in the detoxifying process indicating you are mobilizing and eliminating toxins. Unfortunately, they do not make you feel good.

It is important for someone on the Master Cleanse to know what detox symptoms are and that they usually will go away or be reduced with the next morning's eliminations. The exceptions are headaches due to caffeine withdrawal during the first few days, which may last two to four days, and rashes, which indicate a significant detoxification and may continue for several days. It is next to impossible to go ten consecutive days of cravings or tiredness with no relief in sight, but when you know those feelings will be gone with tomorrow's eliminations, anyone can make it through the Master Cleanse. The Master Cleanse is not about will power. It is about knowledge—what to expect and how to deal with it.

If you had severe symptoms, you might want to consider putting yourself on a health-restoring regimen for several months. Such a regimen should include:

1. Not filling the body with more toxins such as: refined white flour and sugar products, meat, artificial flavors, colors, preservatives, alcohol, tobacco, dairy products, etc.

2. Detoxifying the colon to eliminate the toxins being reabsorbed by the blood and redistributed throughout the entire body. (The Master Cleanse is a way of doing this.)

3. Ensuring the body gets adequate, good (non-tap) water (at least one ounce daily for every two pounds of body weight); non-iodized, unprocessed sea salt; and nutritional, raw vegetables (especially greens), fruits, sprouts, and soaked seeds and nuts to help the body rebuild the depleted nutritional reserves and organs.

4. Removing any stress-producing situations in the current environment.

5. Getting exercise and fresh air by lots of walking.

Now that you know these detox symptoms are only temporary and are milestones that you are becoming healthier, you will have the perspective to complete the cleanse and make it through. After you personally experience the gain you make after a detox day, you will actually begin to look forward to them, knowing that the next day will be a new plateau!

No detox symptoms

Many people wonder if they are eliminating toxins when they have no detox symptoms. The waste comes off in layers. So, you may not see anything happening for days and then have a detox day or see other results. I encourage you to continue through the full ten days. When I did my first cleanse (twenty days) I had nothing but bright yellow liquid for about a week in the middle of the twenty days. Then I had some semi-solid waste and felt great the next day. My wife discovered that just weighing yourself is not a good measure because she found that her body was changing shape and losing inches even when she was not losing weight.

So, measure yourself before you start the cleanse, so you will have something to compare to if your scale is not moving as fast as you want.

Severe detox symptoms

Have you taken a lot of medications? Are you overweight? Do you have allergies? All of these are indications of toxicity. More toxicity means you may have more detox symptoms the first few days relative to others who have less toxins. Sometimes a person is eating a good diet currently, but it is medications they took or an extremely bad diet long before their current cleanse that is causing the symptoms. The solution is to emphasize the elimination part of the Master Cleanse. Drink only six glasses of lemonade, ensure you are doing the laxative tea and salt water flush, drink at least half your weight in lemonade or water each day and take hot soaking baths of at least twenty minutes in two cups of Epsom Salt. If it gets really bad, discontinue the cleanse and use a slower method of detoxifying. (See page 44, "The Detox Diet Scale.") You can always do the cleanse again later. Remember, being healthy is not a one-time event. It is a lifetime process.

"How About Only Five Days? Can We Make a Deal?"

Burroughs says to do the Master Cleanse for at least ten days at a time. Many people have asked if they could do it for less. My experience has shown that the days with the greatest chances for detox symptoms— remember, they are the milestones of progress—are the second, third, seventh and fourteenth (for those that go that long). The second and third days are fairly obvious. That is when the recent waste is being eliminated and thus is causing detox symptoms —cravings, irritability, etc. Notice that the seventh and fourteenth are seven days apart. At a talk given by Victoria Boutenko, a raw vegetarian speaker and writer, she showed a video of a live blood analysis that showed the clumping of red blood cells when people ate cooked food. She said it took seven days for the red blood cells to un-clump. Perhaps there is a seven-day cycle in the body that is triggered by the Master Cleanse. At any rate, I have noticed that the biggest benefits in mental clarity, serenity and focus come for most people after Day 8. The moral of the story? Stick with it for at least ten days, just like Burroughs says.

● The Agitator and the Rinse Cycle

The Master Cleanse is designed to do two things: first to detoxify the body (remove toxins/poisons from the cells and organs in which they are embedded)—The Agitator—and then to eliminate those toxins from the body before they can be reabsorbed and poison the body once again—the Rinse Cycle. Just as a washing machine must incorporate both of those to be effective, so must any good cleanse.

Not eating any solid food permits your body to direct all of its digestive energy toward removing toxins from the cells and organs in which they are embedded. This process is aided by the six to twelve ten-ounce glasses of "lemonade" per day that you will drink on the Master Cleanse. The lemon juice helps to neutralize the acidic wastes and loosen them from where they are stored, and the cayenne pepper increases the blood flow to areas to be detoxified by dilating the blood vessels. The final part of the Agitator is the herbal laxative tea which stimulates the muscular contractions in the intestines, which "agitates" the contents and moves them toward final elimination.

Once the old toxic waste has been mobilized, you need the Rinse Cycle to eliminate it before it is reabsorbed. After the stomach has reduced the food you have eaten to a semi-liquid form, your body pushes it through the intestines where it absorbs what you have given it as nourishment. If the walls of the intestines are coated with years of waste, all daily nutrients must be absorbed through this coating and some of the old putrefied waste is carried into the blood stream.

Sadly, most "civilized" people tend to overeat, and to choose those things which are the most difficult to digest, such as meat and cheese. The final result of this kind of diet over decades is an accumulation of toxic waste, which is then re-absorbed into the blood. (You can read more about this in the excellent books by Dr. Norman W. Walker, such as *Colon Health: The Key to a Vibrant Life*, or *Become Younger*. Dr. Walker, by the way, lived to ninety-nine years of age, was mentally sharp and physically fit throughout his life, and is credited with the statement, "Death begins in the colon.")

The salt water flush is the Rinse Cycle and therefore vital. If you cannot drink the salt water flush in the morning, you should drink the laxative tea both evening and morning. (Take care not to drink more than two cups per day of pure senna tea or four cups per day of tea with 50 percent senna.) However, I believe that the agitator action of the laxative tea is different than the flushing action of the salt water flush and encourage people to do the salt water flush if at all possible. You would not wash your clothes in a washing machine with only an agitator and no rinse cycle, so why clean your digestive tract without a rinse cycle?

● The Master Cleanse Is Not for Everyone

The Master Cleanse is not for everyone. There are some people who should not even attempt it:

- People who are undergoing chemotherapy or have completed chemotherapy within the last six months must not do the Master Cleanse. Chemotherapy is based on the idea that administering a chemical poison will kill cancer cells before healthy cells. Under such treatment, a part of each dose accumulates in the body. (This information is from Max Gerson M.D., who developed a nutritional treatment for tuberculosis, cancer, and other degenerative diseases.) So, many treatments can accumulate a lethal dose if later released all at once. Therefore, such people must use a much slower detox method to avoid liver damage or worse. (See "The Detox Diet Scale" on page 44.)

- People who are recovering from major surgery or a severe wound—we are not talking a cut finger here—should not do the Master Cleanse. In order to build tissue, you must have extra protein. Since the Master Cleanse contains no protein, it will not support massive rebuilding of muscles. There is no danger from this lack of protein for a month or more, but such a lack will slow down healing. If you are recovering from major surgery, ask your surgeon when your healing is complete before doing the cleanse. People not in these categories—recovering from surgery or a severe wound—need not be concerned. People only lose one to two pounds of muscle mass no matter how long they do the cleanse because the body only burns muscle for energy for the first two days for women and three days for men.[3] Thereafter, it only burns fat and waste. This same process explains why athletes on the Master Cleanse do better with walking, jogging and swimming but not weight lifting and bodybuilding.

- Rapidly growing children should not do the Master Cleanse because they need protein for growth. The exception is if they are suffering from asthma or something similar. Several studies have shown fasting to be an effective treatment for such problems for people of all ages.[4]

- Opinion is divided on whether pregnant or nursing women should do the Master Cleanse. I have never heard of a single pregnant or nursing woman to be hurt by the cleanse, but in the spirit of "better safe than sorry," I began to say that pregnant or nursing women should not do the cleanse. Right after I published that in one of my newsletters, I got an email from a midwife who said she had thirty years of experience with the Master Cleanse being done by pregnant and nursing women and no one ever had a problem. Likewise, Stanley Burroughs and another Master Cleanse author, Tom Woloshyn, say that the Master Cleanse is fine for pregnant and nursing mothers. So, I will leave it up to you. (One clever woman, who wanted to lose the extra weight she had gained during pregnancy and was going to be away from her baby for a cruise, stored enough of her breast milk for ten days and did the cleanse while her baby was taken care of by her mother using the stored breast milk.)

There are other people who may not be able to do all ten days of the cleanse. Someone who is much too toxic will find it nearly impossible not to eat. The body has a natural protective mechanism. They will

---

3 Fuhrman, Joel, M.D., *Fasting and Eating for Health*, St. Martin's Griffin, New York, NY, p. 12

4 Papers submitted to the 2001 Fasting Therapy Conference, Ulan Ude, Russian Republic Of Buryatia, Ministry of Public Health Care

go off the cleanse before the detoxification symptoms get to be too much. It is not dangerous for these people to do it, but they will benefit more from the slower methods of detoxification that create less detox symptoms. (See "Detox Diet Scale" on page 44 for a list.)

How do you know if you have a great deal of toxins? If you have two or more of the following, you may be too toxic:

- Allergic to "everything."Alternative medicine equates allergies with toxic reactions. If you are only allergic to bananas, that is probably not too serious. If you are allergic to fifteen things, you need to take it easy.

- Very poor general health

- Multi-year history of strong medical or psychiatric drugs. Antibiotics every few years for infections are probably not much to worry about. Sleeping pills every night for ten years is another situation. If you are on or have had heavy psychiatric drugs, chemotherapy, etc. you should definitely check with your health professional.

- More than seventy pounds overweight. The body stores toxins in fat cells when it runs out of room in the liver. Serious overweight indicates there may be lots of toxins and waste to eliminate.

If you want to try the Master Cleanse even though you have such indicators, please follow the directions given in the next section, "If Detox Symptoms Become Unpleasant."

If you are taking blood thinners or high blood pressure medications, you should do the cleanse in coordination with your prescribing licensed health care practitioner. This is because the Master Cleanse will have similar effects as the medications, so if you are also taking medicine for these issues you may get a double whammy. So, be prepared to have your medication dosage reduced.

If Detox Symptoms Become Unpleasant

1. Drink only the minimum six drinks of lemonade each day.

2. Be sure to drink the herbal laxative tea every evening.

3. Drink enough additional water so that you have drunk at least one ounce of water or lemonade for each two pounds of body weight each day.

4. Be sure to do the salt water flush as given each morning.

5. Take a shower or long, soaking hot bath in two cups of Epsom Salt every day to draw out toxins.

The reasoning behind the recommendations above is to detoxify very lightly, but use the maximum amount of elimination methods so that whatever toxins are mobilized are quickly eliminated before being reabsorbed. Remember, you can do the Master Cleanse several times. So, do not push it.

Headaches

As I pointed out in "Detox Symptoms—The Good, the Bad and the Ugly," people who have heavy daily caffeine habits — coffee, tea, soda with caffeine, etc.— typically have bad headaches when they go cold turkey on the Master Cleanse. Realize it is the caffeine habit you are kicking and persevere. It does not make sense to go off the Master Cleanse in order to attempt to kick the habit without the enhanced elimination procedures. The longest I have known someone to have a headache was four days. Keep in mind if you have a headache for more than a day or so and never had a caffeine habit, this may signal other problems that you should not ignore. Therefore, you should quickly discover the cause.

When It Is Not All Coming Out as Planned ☺

Not having any bowel movements? Here is a checklist to help you.

0. Some people expect they will have black rubbery eliminations on the Master Cleanse. Perhaps they have seen pictures of this on the Internet. This is produced by taking benonite clay and/or psyllium husks, which mechanically push the old wastes out rather than dissolve it. This is not what happens on the Master Cleanse. The lemonade and not eating will dissolve the old waste and toxins. As long as something is coming out, watery or not, do not worry.

1. Are you putting at least two level TEASPOONS of sea salt in the water each morning and having several urgent eliminations within an hour? If this is not happening, you have not got the right amount of salt in the water. For those on a heavy meat and/or cheese diet, it may take two or three days to work, but when you get the amount correct, the result is impossible to miss. You will have no doubt.

2. Are you mixing two tablespoons (one ounce) of fresh squeezed—not bottled—lemon juice into each drink or using these proportions for each batch and only mixing one day at a time?

3. Are you adding cayenne pepper to taste with each drink?

4. Are you drinking one cup of laxative tea each morning as well as each evening and the salt water flush to encourage more elimination? (Note: Discontinue the extra cup in the morning after you get things going.)

5. Are you eating or drinking anything else but lemonade, water, salt water, laxative herb tea and occasional mint tea?

6. Before this cleanse, did you have only one or two BMs per week? Being constipated before the Master Cleanse might mean a little longer before you see results.

7. Are you on any constipating medications? I am NOT suggesting you quit taking any prescribed medications. But they may delay the results of the Master Cleanse.

The Twelve Most Common Pitfalls

More than 25,000 people are members of The Master Cleanse/Raw Food Forum (www.TheMasterCleanse.com) as I write this in March 2012. (More than twenty times that number search through and read it without becoming members.) These twelve pitfalls are the most common. If you can avoid these, you will multiply your chances for success by 12 times.

1. Not getting all the correct written information before starting the cleanse

I know. You think I am saying this just because I want to sell my books. Well, I do want to sell my books. But that is not why I am saying this. Remember the children's game "telephone" where you whisper a message from one person to another? The message starts as "Say, Hi!" and ends as "I am at the post office."

The person who told you how to do it may or may not have remembered all the important information. They may not have the same concerns that you have. So they do not mention something important to you.

There are so many strange alterations. I cannot remember them all. But they have one thing in common. They will not get the great results that everyone else gets by following Stanley Burroughs' instructions. When you verbally tell your friend what you remember about the cleanse, you may be setting them up for a failure. And they may not remember exactly what you said either. I wish I had a dollar for everyone who says, "Oh! two teaspoons of sea salt in the salt water flush. I was trying to do it with two tablespoons!"

I have seen real people on the bulletin board talk about adding soy sauce to the salt water flush so it tastes like soup. (Soy sauce is protein and requires almost as much digestion as hamburger!) Another asked how many of the glasses of orange juice or vegetable soup are permitted each afternoon on the cleanse. (The answer? None!) Another woman talked about how she tried to handle her hunger with vegetable soup each afternoon! (That would start digestion going again and put her back on days two and three, and make her hungry, over and over!)

To really help your friends, either give them the book or tell them to go buy it. They will value it more. And they will get the straight scoop. Their significant other might pick it up and help them or join them, too!

2. Not knowing what "detox" means

"Detox" is short for detoxify — meaning to eliminate toxins (poisons). It comes from "de-" meaning down or away, "toxin" meaning poison, and "-ify" meaning to make or do. So, "detoxify" means to make poisons come out or away (from the body). The toxins in our case are substances that your body can't absorb and use to rebuild the body. They actually harm your body's cells making you fat, tired, irritable, sick or, in extreme cases, dead.

So, when a person detoxifies, or detoxes, she or he is mobilizing the toxins stored in various places and eliminating them. When they are mobilized, the person may become tired, feel pain or aches, be irritable, develop rashes, etc. These symptoms (signs showing that something else exists) tell you that toxins have been mobilized. Next, they need to be eliminated. Once they are eliminated, you will feel better than before. The whole purpose of a cleanse is to eliminate toxins so that you feel better and are healthier than before.

3. Not knowing the detox symptoms

See page 27, "Detox Symptoms—the Good, the Bad and the Ugly."

4. Not knowing that detox symptoms will usually be gone or lessened with the next day's eliminations

Detox symptoms usually go away or at least lessen with the next day's eliminations. This is vital to understand because very few people can make it through ten straight days of cravings. But if you know those feelings will only last one more day, you can make it through all ten days of the Master Cleanse easily.

Too often, I hear of people quitting because they were discouraged and thought nothing was happening. First, their discouragement was a detox symptom — a sign something was happening. Second, they were only one morning away from feeling great and knowing they could do it. So, you can see how important it is to know about this pitfall.

The reverse of this is also important. If you are feeling sick and it doesn't go away or lessen after a few days, it is probably not a detox symptom. What then? If it's serious, consult your licensed health care practitioner. If it's not, either come off the cleanse and handle it or handle it as you think best.

5. Not doing all the elimination actions every day

If you really understand that detoxification is a two step process—mobilized, then eliminated—and that detox symptoms occur when these toxins are mobilized, but not yet eliminated, you will then understand the importance of doing all the elimination actions.

Sometimes a person can neglect one or another elimination action (salt water flush, laxative tea, drinking at least six lemonades a day) for a few days and feel no ill effects. Usually, that comes back to bite them later. Do all the elimination actions every day.

6. Not knowing the worst days are usually two, three and seven

I believe it is important to know which days are going to be the worst. For one thing, you will know that the entire Master Cleanse will not be that difficult. For another, you can look forward to better days. (By the way, people usually gain mental clarity and find that cooking for others does not bother them starting with day eight.)

It is amazing how many people quit on day two, three or seven! (Occasionally someone will be off by a day and have day one be the worst or day six.) In addition to not knowing which days are the worst, they usually do not know the detox symptoms and that they go away if the elimination actions are done each day.

I have observed that the body detoxes in seven-day cycles. When I did my 20-day cleanse, days two, three, seven and fourteen were the worst. I just recently finished a 28-day cleanse, but days 21 and 28 were fine. So, it is not always every seven days, but very frequently it is the case. I have found that each cleanse usually gets easier.

7. Confusing cravings with hunger

How do you tell the difference? If you really want a hamburger, but you would turn down a green salad, it is a craving. Why does it make any difference? When you realize you are feeling cravings, not hunger, you know they are just detox symptoms and will go away the next day.

8. Not drinking more lemonade or water when you feel hungry

Only one person in four reports any hunger on this cleanse. After checking to see if they are craving some food in particular, I tell them to drink more lemonade or water when they feel hungry. And their hunger usually disappears.

9. Eating or drinking anything else except lemonade, salt water, herbal laxative tea or mint tea while on the cleanse (except items prescribed by licensed health professionals)

A lady once posted to The Master Cleanse Bulletin Board that she kept feeling hungry. When I asked her to tell me exactly what she was doing, she told me she was drinking vegetable soup each afternoon! Of course, this was creating new cravings to torture her every day! So, rather than being done with cravings after the third day, she was continuing her cravings every single day of the cleanse!

Other people have asked about taking additional items, such as vitamins, supplements, chewing gum, sweetener for the tea, herbs, etc.

Hundreds of thousands of people have done The Master Cleanse since it was developed by Stanley Burroughs. It works. Just as written. The lemonade and maple syrup have all the necessary vitamins, minerals and calories to support the body for the duration of the cleanse.

10. Not using fresh-squeezed lemon juice

I am not saying you have to freshly squeeze the lemon (or lime) juice for each glass one at a time. If you have to go to work all day, you will have to make up enough for the whole day ahead of time. But try to make the last drink or two with freshly squeezed lemon juice after you get home. By the way, cayenne gets hotter the longer it sits. So, try to make two bottles for the day with three drinks in each bottle and put cayenne in the second bottle just before you are ready to drink it. (Cheap commercial plug: I sell two such bottles in an insulated bag for just this purpose in my web store at www.TheMasterCleanse.com/store.)

Do not use bottled, processed, or yesterday's juice. It is the enzymes (substances that encourage chemical changes) in the lemon juice that make it effective. These enzymes become less effective over time.

By using freshly squeezed juice, your lemonade will be as effective as possible to help dissolve the old waste.

11. Going to social events during the first seven days

Something wonderful happens on day eight. Many people discover that cooking for others becomes much easier. A good friend, after day seven, helped a chef prepare grilled pork tenderloins for dinner and my friend on the cleanse was not bothered at all! (Usually, they gain mental clarity, too.)

However, before then, do not tempt yourself. Especially on days two, three and seven.

12. Being so focused on losing pounds that you do not notice you are losing inches

My wife discovered something interesting. She kept track of her measurements each day as well as her weight. A couple times her weight did not change. But she noticed that she was losing inches in places she wanted. Others talk about being able to fit into clothes they could not wear before even though they had not lost many pounds.

What to Expect Day by Day

These days may be off by one or two. For example, days two and three are usually the worst, but it could be days one and two.

Day 1:

Generally easy. One out of four people has trouble with the salt water flush. If so, you may substitute another cup of herbal laxative tea in the morning for the salt water flush. If you do, try the salt water flush after day seven as it gets easier after you eliminate some mucus. Most people find it much easier on their second or third Master Cleanse. People with caffeine habits may have headaches for the first few days. Four days is the longest I have heard for these headaches. Some people advise quitting caffeine before the cleanse to make it easier, but then you are doing it without the daily "agitator and rinse cycle" of the Master Cleanse which makes quitting easier and faster.

Days 2 and 3:

Usually the worst, although some people have no detox symptoms throughout the cleanse. It is important to remember during these two days that whatever you are feeling, it will lessen or go away with the next morning's eliminations. That is why I think Stanley Burroughs, the developer of the Master Cleanse, was such a genius. Fasting is a great way to rejuvenate the body. However, the toxins that are released can cause a person to feel quite bad. Burroughs added an "agitator and rinse cycle" (laxative tea and salt water flush) to remove toxins quickly so the detox symptoms stay manageable.

For the first two or three days, the body burns muscle for energy. On day three for women and day four for men, the body switches and begins to burn fat and waste for energy. Stick with it because when the body switches over, most people report it is well worth it—calmness, lack of tiredness, clear thinking, and a positive attitude, not to mention losing weight.

Days 4 to 6:

Most people report the benefits mentioned above. This is why I call the Master Cleanse the reset button for the body. Many people report their sense of smell is heightened.

Day 7:

A bit of a detox day, not as bad as days two and three, but possibly some detox symptoms of less intensity. At this point, the cleanse begins to eliminate older waste. These older toxins dissolve like layers of an onion.

Days 7 to 10:

Clear sailing like days four to six. Those who cook for their families generally find that by day eight it does not bother them to prepare food for others. They are beginning to have a sense of detachment from food. Other people find that they no longer are interested in watching TV or playing video games. Perhaps they enjoy soaking in the tub or reading. Many people report their body becoming more flexible, their skin becoming clearer, and less joint pain after this many days of the cleanse.

Day 14:

(if you go that far): Similar to day seven. Detox symptoms of less intensity than those on days two and three.

Day 16:

Some people experience a calm detachment toward food and life as well as a chance to reevaluate goals and plans. I discovered an intense desire to watch the Food Channel and smell other people's food, but I was not tempted to eat any of it—kind of like a Scratch 'n Sniff!

Days 21, 28, 35, etc.:

In my experience, I found detox days came every seven days or so. Sometimes I would be surprised by a solid elimination and would be amazed as I had not eaten anything for weeks!

The Detox Diet Scale

If you bring toxins out of storage faster than your body can neutralize and eliminate them, you will get a detox symptom or reaction. This is because the toxins can be reabsorbed before they are neutralized and eliminated.

The Master Cleanse is the second fastest method of detoxification. (A water-only fast is the fastest.) However, faster is not always better because it may be more than the body can handle. People with poor elimination or people with too many toxins need a slower method so their elimination system can keep up. In the case of those on or just off chemotherapy, this may possibly even cause harm.

I know a lady in New York who had a several-year history of strong medical drugs and was surprised that she was doing so well on the Master Cleanse until I discovered that she was using bottled, and thus pasteurized, lemon juice. (Pasteurization kills enzymes and severely reduces the effectiveness of the lemon juice.)

When she tried fresh-squeezed lemon juice, she had much stronger detox symptoms and had to switch to a slower method of detoxification. (By the way, this incident convinced me that bottled lemon juice is not acceptable for the Master Cleanse.)

Here is my scale of detoxifying actions ranked from fastest (1) to slowest (10). The fastest methods are good so long as you can tolerate the detox symptoms. If they are more than you can endure, see the section above "If Detox Symptoms Become Unpleasant" for actions you can take to reduce them for fast relief. If you still cannot handle them, switch to a slower method.

1. Pure-water fast (if done for more than a couple days, it is best done under a doctor's supervision)

2. The Master Cleanse, which permits working and aerobic exercise (as opposed to the pure-water fast, which sometimes requires bed rest.) Note: Bodybuilding exercise is not compatible with the Master Cleanse as there is no protein. You can live without protein for 40 days or longer, but you cannot build muscles without protein.

3. Fruit juice fast (fruits are detoxifiers)

4. Vegetable juice fast (veggies build up the body with vitamins, proteins and minerals)

5. Enemas or colonics (can be combined with all these other methods *except* the Master Cleanse)

6. 100 percent raw vegan diet

7. Predominantly raw vegan diet with the rest of the diet being cooked vegetarian food

8. 100 percent vegetarian diet without sugar or artificially preserved, colored, flavored, sweetened, or prepared foods

9. Drinking a green smoothie every day for breakfast. (Go to www.TheMasterCleanse.com/topic/raw-food-recipes/ for the recipe.

10. Soaking in a hot Epsom Salt bath (two cups to a regular sized tub) at least three times a week for twenty minutes, which can also be combined with any of the above.

Part III
Can I Ask You A Question?

Acid/alkaline balance/pH?

Much attention has been focused lately on alkalizing the body. The need for this can be clearly seen when you realize that meat, sugar, flour, and cooked foods produce acid in the body when digested. Raw fruits, vegetables, seeds and some nuts produce an alkaline condition. This includes lemons, which are acid before they are eaten, but produce an alkaline result when eaten. When you fast, the body begins to mobilize and eliminate the acidic toxins. Therefore the urine pH during a fast becomes acidic. Calcium, magnesium, potassium and sodium (alkaline minerals) are used by the liver to neutralize the acidic toxins before they are eliminated. This is the reason you have to have alkaline mineral reserves to do the Master Cleanse. After the cleanse, the body is in more of an alkaline state.

Adding anything to the MC

Can I add a colon cleanser?

As to whether psyllium, bentonite clay, herbs or colon cleansers are the only way to remove old waste on the colon walls, I go by the appearance of the tongue. Chinese doctors have used the tongue to diagnose internal organs for thousands of years and I am amazed at what it reveals during the cleanse! When I checked tongue color, I discovered that the two people I know who have eaten a pure raw veggie, fruit, nut and seed diet have perfectly pink tongues. I have also produced a perfectly pink tongue after adding an ounce of wheatgrass juice to my raw food diet for seven days right after a seventeen-day cleanse. Based on that, I would say that colon cleanses, psyllium, etc. are not the only way to remove old waste on your colon walls. Not only does the MC cleanse the colon, it also gives the colon and digestive system a rest to rejuvenate. So, stick to the program as developed to get the best results.

Hi Peter, I just have to send a note, and should've done it sooner, but was just thinking about it. I did the Master Cleanse for 31 days (waited till my tongue turned pink again) this spring. I had never felt better! The amount of energy was endless, and I felt awesome!! On top of feeling great, I lost 80 lbs!! I couldn't believe it when I started trying on my clothes! Thank you so much for sharing this incredible information!!

N.S.
Plattsmouth, NE
September 30, 2008

Can I take mineral supplements?

The maple syrup, cayenne and lemon provide all the minerals needed for daily function and cleansing. The lemon also acts as a blood alkalizer. I recommend you follow the cleanse as written and abstain from any supplements until after the cleanse. *The Master Cleanser* by Stanley Burroughs says you do not need and should not take any supplements while on the cleanse.

Adding anything to the MC

When one of our cleansers tried adding wheat grass tablets on the evening of Day 4, he cancelled them on the evening of Day 6 as his irritable bowel flared up. That seems to confirm what Burroughs says about not needing supplements on the cleanse.

Can I take vitamins, shakes or protein?

Fasting is what gives the Master Cleanse its power. Fasting has been used for thousands of years to rejuvenate the body and focus the mind. Jesus, Moses, Ghandi, Buddha, Mohammed, Socrates, Plato, and Hippocrates (The Father of Western Medicine) all fasted and recommended fasting. Allan Cott, MD, wrote *Fasting: The Ultimate*

Diet, a million-copy bestseller, in 1975 on the benefits of fasting. So, adding anything reduces its effectiveness. Stick to the program as developed by Stanley Burroughs to get the best results. This does NOT mean discontinue any PRESCRIBED medications.

What about prescription meds?

Do not discontinue anything prescribed by a licensed healthcare practitioner without at least getting a second opinion. Remember, there are many kinds of licensed healthcare practitioners: chiropractors, naturopaths, acupuncturists, doctors of oriental medicine, nutritionists, etc. If you are on medication for high blood pressure, know that fasting has been scientifically shown to reduce blood pressure. So, you will very likely have to adjust your dosage. In the same way, those on blood thinners should know that cayenne pepper acts as a blood thinner, which may require adjusting dosages as well. Anyone on chemotherapy or anti-depressants should see those topics.

Additional Benefits—A reset button for the body

Not only does the Master Cleanse make the body healthier, it also temporarily gives peace of mind and a sense of peaceful energy. My first cleanse was for twenty days. I have also done this cleanse for two and three days. Burroughs is right about doing it for at least ten days. The real gains start after Day 7, which is usually a day with noticeable detox symptoms. A twenty-day cleanse produced, for me and many others, temporary spiritual gains beyond just health. This cleanse is like pressing reset for the body. It puts everything back to normal.

After the cleanse

Craving bad food after the MC

First, take probiotics when you resume eating solid food. Follow the directions on the label. It will help prevent cravings. Then if you want meat or dairy, go ahead but include a salad meal each day as well. You can always do another cleanse. A fellow I met told me he had done the cleanse three times. After the first, he was no longer interested in red meat. After the second cleanse, he found he liked raw vegetables more. After the third, he was no longer interested in meat and wanted organic vegetables. That covered three years of his life.

Gas or digestive problems?

If you have gas or digestive problems, you should continue the cleanse for a few more days.

Healthy diet after the MC?

Breakfast should be the MC lemonade. In addition, eat a salad every day as well and primarily eat raw fruit, vegetables, seeds, nuts and berries.

Lemonade or salt water flush after the MC?

The salt water flush may be done after the MC whenever you feel it will help. Be sure to do it on an empty stomach, though. The MC lemonade is recommended as a daily breakfast drink.

No BMs after the MC?

Generally, it takes two days before most people have BMs again after the MC because there is nothing in the colon during the Master Cleanse. If you still are not eliminating, be sure to take probiotics when you return to solid food as probiotics make up 30% of the bulk of eliminations. Also, daily green smoothies in the morning promote eliminations as well due to the fibers in the greens.

Will I gain the weight back?

To prevent weight coming back, be sure you eat at least 50% fresh raw vegetables and fruit and if you do eat meat or dairy, do a salt water flush the next day. In addition, I recommend doing the Master Cleanse at least twice a year. Weight gain is all about what you eat. If you eat foods that your body sees as toxins, the body will protect itself by making mucus to line the digestive tract and store the toxins in the body fat. That is just how it is. Eat junk and get fat. If you eat real food, nutritious food, you will lose to an ideal weight and not gain it back at all. There you go: Total control of your weight and health!

EXACTLY what I've been looking for for years!!! I'm 36, female, and was 50 lbs. overweight according to my family doctor's chart. I learned about the Master Cleanse from watching a makeover show and Robin Quivers was featured. I began the cleanse THE next day! I lost 15 lbs in 15 days and haven't gained it back! ... I'm doing the MC for the second time and am looking forward to losing the final 35 pounds, having fantastic energy and feeling great!!

S. N.
California
October 28, 2004

Agave nectar vs. maple syrup

I had a phone call from a lady who told me she had done a Master Cleanse with agave and didn't feel like it had done as much as maple syrup and wanted to do the MC again with maple syrup. When I researched it, I discovered that it has to be heated to approximately 140 degrees to cause it to become sweet. (It is not sweet naturally.) That causes it to be about 85% fructose, which makes it higher in fructose (42–55%) than high fructose corn syrup (HFCS). HFCS was linked to obesity and liver problems in a 2007 study by Brent Tetri, M.D., professor of internal medicine at Saint Louis University Liver Center presented at the Digestive Diseases Week conference in 2007. Maple syrup is about 2% fructose. In addition, agave contains about a third of the potassium in a similar amount of maple syrup. I also know that Tom Woloshyn, who also wrote a book about the Master Cleanse, discourages people from using agave for the Master Cleanse and cites another practitioner who discourages people from using agave for more than ten days because it led to demineralization.

Anti-depressants

It is not advisable to take yourself off anti-depressants without proper medical/professional assistance. For assistance, I recommend going to www.TheRoadBack.org. They have a free book on how to come off anti-depressants safely and a list of doctors if you need more help. I do not recommend doing the cleanse if you are on a strong anti-depressant. They are very toxic and can create severe detox symptoms during the cleanse.

Artificial sweeteners

For goodness sake, don't use any artificial sweeteners in your tea while on the Master Cleanse. Even after the cleanse, I would recommend dropping them. There are numerous studies on their ill effects.

Beyond 10 days—Can I go longer than 10 days?

I would divide the benefits of going beyond the tenth day into two categories. The first are spiritual in nature. Although temporary, I found a sense of serenity, an increased ability to face and handle problems, the ability to face stress without handling it with food, seeing your life goals in perspective and the absence of a desire to eat "bad" food even while I could appreciate and enjoy the smell of it. The idea of consuming something that would be bad for my body even though it smelled good was like the idea of eating a scratch n' sniff sticker. You would not even think of it. The second category of gain is physical improvement. I will tell you that people I know who have done more than twenty days, say the benefits came from the additional days.

Boredom

Boredom is one of the detox symptoms. When you get past the first two or three days, you will feel wonderful. That is your natural state. Boredom is the result of toxins in your body.

Bowel Movements, eliminations

Hot/burning BMs

The burning bowel movements are caused by the toxins leaving your body. Toxins are acid. They burn.

No BMs on the MC

Some people may be taking medicines and many of them make a person constipated as a side effect. Sometimes it takes a few days.

1. People who eat SAD (the Standard American Diet of 100% meat, dairy, cooked food, no raw vegetables, and very few raw fruits) get "plugged up" and it can take two or three days before the full quart salt water flush begins to eliminate.

2. Not drinking at least six ten-ounce drinks of lemonade a day (or more for larger people) makes for less eliminations.

3. The salt water flush not only produces several liquid eliminations starting within thirty to sixty minutes, but also provides the colon with liquid to promote later eliminations and make them easier.

So, be patient, ensure you are doing the laxative tea at night and the salt water flush in the morning, and drink six to twelve lemonades with fresh lemon juice as instructed. Then if you still are not eliminating, add a single cup of laxative tea first thing in the morning as well. Beyond that, don't worry. The cleanse will work it out, believe me.

By the way, some people think if they eliminate only a bright yellow liquid that it doesn't count as a bowel movement. I consider anything that comes out the "back end" as a bowel movement.

Watery/runny BMs

Liquid BMs are the usual on the cleanse. Solid ones are unusual after the first day, although you could have semi-solid ones on later days because the intestines detox in layers. Therefore you will have periods of runny BMs and possibly semi-solid ones later. The waste of a lifetime comes off in layers and takes quite a while to dissolve if you have been eating a diet heavy in meat and dairy. But don't worry, the cayenne and lemon juice WILL dissolve it.

Yellow BMs

I believe the yellow is from bile. It is true that B12 and other B vitamins turn your pee yellow, but I have never seen them turn BMs yellow.

Breaking the Master Cleanse

The longer you are on the MC, the more important it is to break it correctly. People who have only been on it for only two or three days generally have no problem breaking it, provided they drink orange juice for the first day after they stop drinking lemonade. After ten days, you should follow the procedure for breaking the cleanse because going straight back to food can make you nauseous and/or cause stomach pain. After seventeen days, correctly breaking the Master Cleanse is important and after thirty or more days it is VERY important. I did it wrong once and had nausea and stomach pains for more than an hour. Here are the Instructions for breaking it:

For vegetarians: Slowly drink several glasses of orange juice for each of the first two days. You may dilute the juice if you like or have any digestive problems. On the third day, drink orange juice in the morning, eat fresh fruit for lunch and have a fruit or raw vegetable salad for dinner.

For non-vegetarians: Slowly drink several glasses of orange juice for the first day and through the afternoon of the second. You may dilute the juice if you like or have any digestive problems. For dinner on the second day, drink mostly the broth of a vegetable soup you make yourself that afternoon from several different vegetables, such as carrots, celery, potatoes, onions, tomatoes, green peppers, zucchini, beans, peas, lentils, etc. No meat or meat stock. You may add rice, dehydrated veggies or spices, but use sea salt sparingly. The less you cook the soup, the better. You may have rye wafers with the soup, but not bread or crackers. Make enough for lunch the next day. On the third day, drink orange juice in the morning. Have the rest of the soup for lunch. For dinner, eat whatever vegetarian salads, vegetables or fruit you wish.

I just finished doing the MC for 11 days and it was pretty easy. I didn't feel so hungry as I missed eating. I lost only about 8 lbs, but I didn't really need to lose weight to begin with.

I broke the fast by the book. Fresh squeezed organic OJ. The second day I had OJ and I made a delicious soup. Yummy yummy. I sauteed some onions and garlic in a bit of olive oil, then added some chopped kambocha squash, parsnips, carrots, potatoes, and sauteed for a bit longer. I added some rosmary, thyme, a pinch of salt and some cayyane pepper and a bit of water and sauteed some more. Then I added about a quart of water and some red lentles and cooked for about 30 mintutes.

On day 2 I had some broth for lunch and a bit of the soup for dinner. I am happy to report that I had my first BM this morning (day three after). Mostly, I am just craving fruit and raw vegetables. Normally, I would be craving pizza, but one of the reasons I did this was to give me a jump start on eating well, and it worked.

A.L.
Brooklyn, NY
April 20, 2006

Bronchitis, asthma

In Germany, Japan and Russia, there are annual medical conferences on the benefits of fasting. The 2000 Russian conference heard papers citing the benefits of fasting for treating ten different diseases including asthma, bronchitis, hypertension (high blood pressure), viral lung infections and obesity.

Unexpected results! ... The cleanse wasn't easy but was successful, even in a way I hadn't expected. After 4 or 5 days I realized that my allergies/hay fever/asthma symptoms were greatly diminished and so I quit taking any medication (even over the counter.) Stayed on the cleanse for 14 days and did not have any symptoms for those days or 2 months following. Did my second 14 day cleanse after 3 months (with symptoms returning) with the same results. Am really trying to watch what I eat now in hopes of keeping all the sneezing, runny nose and eyes, and breathing problems at bay.

A.
September 29, 2007

Brushing your teeth on the MC

I see no reason not to brush your teeth. Just don't use toothpaste with artificial flavors, colors, preservatives sweeteners or fluoride. (Fluoride is so poisonous that swallowing any more than a pea-sized amount of fluoride toothpaste requires calling a poison control center! See the warning on your tube of toothpaste. Our government has now persuaded two-thirds of the country to add it to drinking water. Instead, it should be removed from our drinking water!) During the cleanse, I don't use any toothpaste. Use mint tea to help handle mouth and body odors. By the way, if you are going for a clear, pink tongue as a sign of the cleanse being complete, check your tongue 24 hours after brushing it.

Candida/yeast

The Master Cleanse is not a guaranteed cure for candida/yeast. It does work for some and it doesn't work for others. People who have candida before are likely to have it after. My basis for these remarks is a poll that has been running on my website forum since October 2006 that has responses from 193 people.

Cayenne pepper

Cayenne pepper acts as the accelerator pedal for the cleanse. It dilates blood vessels, increasing circulation. It feeds the heart, is a great source of Vitamin C, and breaks down mucus & old waste. So, don't skip the cayenne. Also, don't take cayenne in capsules. According to Dr. Richard Schulze, a master herbalist, people who take cayenne capsules do not receive much of the benefit of the cayenne. The nerve endings in the mouth respond almost instantly to send blood throughout the body. This whole process is missed if you take capsules. Also, gelatin is made from boiled skin, bones and tendons. That is a lot of digestive work—especially when you are not eating to give your digestive system a rest. So, taking cayenne capsules should not be done.

Do not put so much in that you hate the taste of the lemonade and then don't drink it. However, do try to stretch your tolerance of it. Not getting enough cayenne will definitely slow down your cleanse. If you don't like it or are not used to spicy heat, start with a sprinkle of cayenne and gradually increase it as you learn to like it. It is a learned food.

There are three things that will make cayenne hotter: 1) Mixing a whole day's batch and putting cayenne in the drink when you make it. Cayenne gets stronger the longer it sits in the drink. 2) Not shaking or stirring the container before drinking. This is especially true if you work and make several glasses at once. The cayenne will sink to the bottom and the last sips will be very, very hot. 3) There are several strengths of cayenne. The common one sold in supermarkets is usually 30,000 heat units. Health food stores also carry that kind and sometimes another hotter one, African Bird Pepper.

It is such a wonderful herb. I want to share a great web page explaining its virtues: www.shirleys-wellness-cafe.com/cayenne.htm

Cheating

I am assuming that you cheated on Day 2, 3 or 7 as those are usually the ones with the most cravings and detox symptoms. Don't beat yourself up! You took a step forward and did something good for your body. Take pride in the initial step.

Next, check whether you followed the directions in the book exactly. Herbal laxative tea at night, salt water flush every morning, six to twelve ten-ounce drinks of lemonade in the right proportions each day and nothing else except water or perhaps mint tea? If not, you made it tougher on yourself by not eliminating the toxins you are mobilizing. If so, they were just reabsorbed and you had stronger detox symptoms. If that was the case, it was just as well that you went off what you thought was "the Master Cleanse."

Think of cleansing and diet as a lifelong process, not as a one-time event. You don't get a cleansing report card and then go on to other things in life. You learn about you and your body and how the two of you need to get along. Work toward eating more raw vegetables, fruits, nuts, and seeds. Have some fresh juices. Do the Master Cleanse again. The urgent desire to eat something else, anything else, and the desire just to CHEW something are both detox symptoms that will pass with the next elimination or two.

I'm starting my 2nd round of the Master Cleanse diet. The 1st time was 1.5 years ago. I did it for 20 days and lost 22 lbs. I cheated 3x (once a week) during this period and still lost the weight. I don't recall what the last two cheats were, but the 1st one was a cheeseburger from a fast food place. It wasn't that I was hungry, it was just food lust. I was never hungry on the diet.

I gained back what I'd lost and then some, but I didn't exercise back then and my job was very hectic at the time and eating right and exercising just wasn't in the cards. It was work/ sleep/work and so on for a very long time.

I started again on Monday, and Tuesday night I cheated (Jumbo Jack from Jack in the box). But I was working late, didn't bring enough lemonade to work late, so I was starving.

I am exercising this time around. 3-5x a week, and once a week with a trainer. I told him that I'm going back on this diet. He hadn't heard of it, but he will be surprised in a few weeks when I jump back on the scale for him at the gym and I'm quite a bit lighter. Also, I remember last time after a few days, I had more energy. Why not utilize that extra energy in the gym to burn off more weight?

Last time was 20 days. I may do 25 or 30 this time (especially since I already cheated at the beginning of this cleanse and I want to see what will happen with less cheating).

P.M.
September 8, 2006

Chemotherapy

If you have been on chemotherapy less than six months ago, do not do the MC. If you have been on chemotherapy more than six months ago, you should consult a licensed healthcare practitioner before starting the cleanse. (Max Gerson, MD, [www.gerson.org] reported that anywhere between 20%–40% of each dose of chemotherapy medicine is stored in the body and could be released during detoxification.) Then, if you decide to do the cleanse considering you have had chemo, I would just "stick a toe in the water" and only drink the minimum six drinks of lemonade each day. I would also be sure to take the herbal laxative tea in the evening and drink at least one ounce of water or lemonade for each two pounds of your body weight each day. Be sure to do the salt water flush as given each morning, and take long, soaking hot baths with Epsom salts to draw out toxins. (Do not do this in fluoridated water! Fluoride is more toxic than lead and a serious enzyme inhibitor. Cancer patients and survivors must avoid drinking, bathing or showering in fluoridated water.) The reason for these warnings is that you want to detoxify these residual toxins with a maximum of elimination. So that whatever toxins are loosened/mobilized will be quickly eliminated.

Also, I would immediately discontinue the cleanse if any detox symptoms didn't disappear or lessen with the next day's eliminations or if you are feeling bad on Day 4. Under those circumstances, discontinue the cleanse and use one of the slower methods of detoxification on the Detox Diet Scale. Even then, you may have to eat some cooked rice or bread to slow down the raw food detoxification depending on symptoms. You can always do the Master Cleanse next year, so don't try to push it.

Chewing gum

Chewing gum consists of five main ingredients: a gum base, sugar, corn syrup, softeners and flavorings. Some gums include artificial chemicals to sweeten them. These have to be handled by the body as toxins. The idea is to give the digestive and elimination organs a rest so they can use their energy to cleanse and rejuvenate. Don't chew gum.

Chills—feeling cold

Any sort of fasting lowers metabolism and that means the body is colder. The Master Cleanse fits right in there. By the way, the idea that you want to have fast metabolism so you can eat a lot has a darker side. As detailed by Joel Fuhrman, MD in his book *Eat to Live*, a slower metabolism can lead to extended lifespan if you eat the right (vegetarian) foods.

Cleansing length—Why 10 days? Can I do less?

Burroughs says to do the cleanse for a minimum of ten days. He doesn't say why, but here are my thoughts. Days 2 and 3 are generally the worst because the body hasn't yet switched to burning fat (scientifically called going into ketosis). Day 7 is the first time old waste is eliminated. So, doing it for three days or less is feeling unpleasant with no actual old waste eliminated. At least eliminate some of the old waste and give yourself a few days of really enjoying the feeling of energy and happiness. That is ten days.

Colonics

I have done colonics before my first Master Cleanse and after it and I did an herbal cleanse after the first MC just to see the difference. I have found the Master Cleanse is the best for me and have no need for colonics. Others I have talked to like colonics and have done them after the Master Cleanse. I think it comes back to the waste accumulating in layers in the colon. There are many years of waste in most people's colons and that takes several Master Cleanses or several series of colonics. Although Burroughs warns against colonics and says they only clean out the last few feet of the colon (good point), the choice to use them is a personal one. The one thing I know with great certainty is that people's bodies are different and respond differently to treatment.

Cooking for others

Many people discover around Day 8 that cooking for others becomes much easier. A good friend, after Day 7, helped a chef prepare grilled pork tenderloins for dinner and my friend on the cleanse wasn't bothered at all!

Cramping—Abdominal & menstrual cramps

For those who suffer from unexplainable cramping, here is something to try. After reading the website on the benefits of cayenne pepper, one of our cleansers tried this, and it worked immediately. She took a little more than one-half teaspoon of cayenne, put it on the back of her tongue. She then took a drink of lemonade. The cramping stopped instantly! She also had to eliminate immediately afterwards. It was like a miracle. It also worked for her on menstruation cramps.

Detox symptoms

Aches/pains, nausea, vomiting

A few people on the Master Cleanse get headaches or other aches, in my experience perhaps 5% or less. Those who get headaches usually had a caffeine habit (coffee or soft drinks) before starting on the Master Cleanse. Detoxifying from caffeine with the Master Cleanse with the salt water flush and laxative tea is probably much easier than going off it "cold turkey." Caffeine headaches are usually one or two days.

The most I have heard of are four days. Persist. Nausea and vomiting are much rarer, but not unheard of. Again these are detox symptoms and will go away.

Other people may have aches and pains from previous illnesses for a few days before these aches and pains disappear a few days later. A friend had very severe hemorrhoids prior to the Master Cleanse. They appeared a few days after he started and went away a few days later. It was his impression that they would not be back.

It's working for me! I bought this book about the Master Cleanse about 1 1/2 yrs. ago. I only made the third day. This time I'm on my 7th. I only experienced a few times with nausea and twice thought I had hunger pains. Drinking another lemonade helped with that. I really wasn't sure I would make it but now I'm sure of it. I lost 7 lbs. so far and my clothes fit better. It wasn't for the weight, I did this, but to cleanse and prepare to start eating better. It has cleared the congestion in my chest. I hope it helps with the many other health issues. My husband stopped on the 4th day, but the first day, he dropped 6.5 lbs. and a couple of lbs. each day after. That was a lot of liquid retention to be carrying around his heart and lungs. One of my daughter's completed this summer and it made her feel so much better. She's eating healthier now and still losing weight...looks great. I feel better too!

L.S.
September 25, 2007

Burning bowel movements

Toxins and other waste are acidic. I have found that when I eliminate old waste and other toxins, my bowel movements are actually hot. During my first Master Cleanse, my eliminations actually burned. I have also noticed that when I have serious detox symptoms as listed above, my eliminations the next morning are typically hot. This may be so bad in the first few days that you need to put some Vitamin E oil on your butt to soothe it. It acts within minutes.

Occasionally, someone will ask if it is the cayenne that burns. While cayenne in large quantities can temporarily cause hot bowel movements, this does not explain how—on a constant dose of cayenne—one can suddenly experience hot bowel movements after several days of normal temperatures. No, I am convinced it is the acidic toxins being eliminated.

Cravings

When your body is detoxifying from ribs, hamburgers, pizza, cheese, etc., you will crave whatever is being detoxified. Paavo Airola discusses this concept on page 153 of his book *How to Get Well*.

Irritability, boredom, etc.

The irritability of dieters is common knowledge. Among the reasons for this is that reduced eating allows the body to detox and one of the symptoms of detoxification is irritability. In this class of symptoms, I also include boredom, anxiety, wanting to "just chew something," and wanting to quit the Master Cleanse. It is quite remarkable how the next day's eliminations can change your attitude toward the Master Cleanse.

When you get to Day 8 or so, you may discover for yourself that your natural mood is positive and cheerful. I have a friend in Georgia who told me how surprised he was that he was able to stay so upbeat during the Master Cleanse in the face of some serious problems.

Tiredness

It should not be strange that the toxins which age you and drain your energy should make you tired. They only do that until they are eliminated. That is why both the herbal laxative tea and salt water flush are so important. They are the "Agitator" and "Rinse Cycle" of the Master Cleanse. Most people have a day or two when they feel tired. Give yourself permission to rest on those days.

What are detox symptoms?

Detox symptoms are what you feel when toxins are mobilized, but not yet eliminated. I divide detox symptoms into five classes as given below.

1. Cravings

2. Irritability, boredom, etc.

3. Headaches, other aches & pains, rashes

4. Tiredness

5. Burning bowel movements

In medicine, these are called Herxheimer Reactions. In alternative medicine, they are called detox symptoms or healing crises. They are a double-edged sword. Detox symptoms are a milestone in the detoxifying process indicating you are mobilizing and eliminating toxins. Unfortunately, they do not make you feel good.

It is important for someone on the Master Cleanse to know what detox symptoms are and that they usually will go away or be reduced with the next morning's eliminations. The exceptions are headaches due to caffeine withdrawal during the first few days, which may last two to four days, and rashes, which indicate a significant detoxification and may continue for several days. It is next to impossible to go ten consecutive days of cravings or tiredness with no relief in sight, but when you know those feelings will be gone with tomorrow's eliminations, anyone can make it through the Master Cleanse. The Master Cleanse is not about will power. It is about knowledge—what to expect and how to deal with it.

If your problems don't lessen or go away after a few days off the cleanse, consult a licensed healthcare practitioner. If the symptoms do go away, you might want to consider putting yourself on a health-restoring regimen for several months. I believe such a regimen should include:

1) Not filling the body with more toxins as found in: refined white flour and sugar products, meat, artificial flavors, colors, preservatives, alcohol, tobacco, dairy products, etc.

2) Detoxifying the colon to eliminate the toxins being reabsorbed by the blood and redistributed throughout the entire body. (The Master Cleanse is a way of doing this.)

3) Ensuring the body gets adequate, good (non-tap) water (at least one ounce daily for every two pounds of body weight); non-iodized, unprocessed sea salt; and nutritional, raw vegetables (especially greens), fruits, sprouts, and soaked seeds and nuts to help the body rebuild the depleted nutritional reserves and organs.

4) Removing any stress-producing situations in the current environment.

5) Getting exercise and fresh air by lots of walking.

> It sure worked for me! I read Peter's book and did the cleanse with great success! As I did the cleanse, I already knew what to expect because it was covered so well in his book. Knowing about the detox symptoms and why I would feel good one day and bad the next, kept me going. Knowing which days were likely to be the worst was invaluable! ... I also bought and read *The Master Cleanser* by Stanley Burroughs and am so glad I read Peter's book also. Burroughs' book didn't mention the five classes of detox symptoms, which days are usually the worst, or have answers to the numerous questions I and others had. I was impressed that Peter kept the actual procedure of the Master Cleanse/Lemonade Diet exactly as Stanley Burroughs wrote it and gave full credit to Stanley Burroughs. It's nice to see someone that caring and honest. Burroughs book was the first, but I liked the simplicity and reading ease of Peter's book.
>
> J.L.
> Ozarks
> May 9, 2005

No detox symptoms

Many people wonder if they are eliminating toxins when they have no detox symptoms. The waste comes off in layers. So, you don't see anything happening for days and then have a detox day and see some results. I encourage you to continue through the full ten days. When I did my first cleanse (twenty days) I had nothing but bright yellow liquid for about a week in the middle of the twenty days. Then I had some semi-solid waste and felt great the next day. My wife discovered that just weighing yourself is not a good measure because she found that her body was changing shape and losing inches even when she was not losing weight.

Severe detox symptoms

Have you taken a lot of medications? Are you overweight? Do you have allergies? All of these are indications of toxicity. More toxicity means the first few days may have more detox symptoms relative to others who aren't in that condition. Sometimes a person is eating a good diet currently, but it is medications they took or an extremely bad diet long before their current cleanse that is causing the symptoms. The solution is to emphasize the elimination part of the Master Cleanse. Drink only six glasses of lemonade, ensure you are doing the laxative tea and salt water flush, drink at least half your weight in lemonade or water each day and take hot soaking baths of at least twenty minutes in two cups of Epsom Salt. If it gets really bad, discontinue the cleanse and use a slower method of detoxifying. You can always do the cleanse again later. Remember, getting healthy is not a one-time event. It is a lifetime process.

I had bad allergies and sinus problems prior to my first MC in March. By day 8 on my MC I developed a bad sinus infection, fever and everything, but I stuck through it and ended my cleanse on day 13. [Since the MC] I have not had a sinus infection or serious allergy problems—even in Atlanta with its ridiculous pollen count.

P.B.
Arlanta, GA
March 14, 2006

Detoxification—What is it?

Detoxification is the process of removing toxins from the body. It is not done in a single step. Toxins do not just disappear. There are two steps. First, the toxins have to be mobilized from wherever they are stored—mostly in fat cells, but also in the joints and other places. (The body stores these toxins mainly in fat cells to protect itself rather than let them circulate.) Second they are neutralized by the liver and eliminated through the colon, kidneys, lungs and skin. Many people are not aware that their skin is part of the elimination system of their bodies. Normally, the body can handle detoxification without major changes to the skin. However, when there are more toxins than can be easily eliminated by the liver, kidneys, colon and lungs, the skin will break out in a rash. You might say the detoxification system has been thrown into "overdrive" to handle the increased load. This is why allergies are regarded as signs of increased toxic load on the body by some alternative medical practitioners.

You can see your detoxification progress by watching your tongue. By the second day, your tongue will become coated. The coat will increase for the first week or so and then gradually disappear and your tongue will begin to turn clear and pink from the edges in toward the center and the tip toward the back of the tongue. The best indication that your cleanse is complete is when your tongue is entirely clean and pink. This took me twenty days on my first cleanse. My tongue goes through this same cycle of getting coated and then going back to clear and pink each time I cleanse.

When your tongue becomes clear and pink, chances are that your skin will begin to glow because it is no longer being forced to eliminate as many toxins as before. People who are on Day 8 or later frequently hear compliments on their complexion.

I ended up doing the cleanse for 20 days (my goal was to go until my tongue turned pink), and I went through many ups and downs and periods of wanting to quit. But I finished, and will use this tool periodically for the rest of my life. My energy was amazing (I planted a garden and repainted my kitchen, by myself!), and the satisfaction I had when I was done, from being able to see it through to the end, was more than I can explain. Anyone who wants to take control of their health truly should try this fast. It is amazing, and you will learn much about yourself.

J.T.
Rapid City, SD
September 25, 2007

Diabetes

I have had a number of people with diabetes ask about doing the Master Cleanse. In *Healing for the Age of Enlightenment,* Burroughs instructs diabetics to use only a bare tablespoon of molasses in the lemonade at first while decreasing the amount of insulin slightly. Then each day gradually increase the amount of molasses while decreasing the amount of insulin, regularly checking the sugar level in the urine and blood to ensure it is within normal range. When you reach two tablespoons of molasses and the insulin has been eliminated, switch to two tablespoons of organic Grade B maple syrup instead of molasses. Upon completing the Master Cleanse, a diet of fresh raw vegetables, nuts, seeds and fruits is recommended as Burroughs describes diabetes as the result of nutritional deficiencies due to a white sugar and white flour diet. Before following these instructions you should consult with your licensed healthcare practitioner.

I am an insulin-dependant diabetic and have been for 26 years. I did this cleanse with intense monitoring of my blood sugar, with no ill effects. I had low blood sugar only once. My insulin intake was reduced by more than half after 3 days. I realize it will now increase, but not to where it was before I started. The best thing is that I now have all of this new-found energy and will be utilizing it to work out 5 or 6 days a week now. Not to mention my eating habits are going to change dramatically as well. I will say that I would only recommend the cleanse to a diabetic who really knows their body well!!

R.

● Diarrhea

Is it actually diarrhea or just four or five watery bowel movements from the salt water? Diarrhea lasts all day. The salt water flush only produces eliminations for an hour or so starting thirty to sixty minutes after you drink the salt water. If it is really diarrhea, discontinue the laxative tea and salt water until the diarrhea is gone. Your body is getting rid of wastes. If the diarrhea continues for more than three days, discontinue the cleanse. Eating grated raw apples or cooked white rice generally stops diarrhea. If that doesn't stop it, you should see a licensed healthcare practitioner since diarrhea can be serious if it continues for a long time.

Emotional detox

I have had plenty of "emotional detox days" and so have others. One lady had a dream that resolved an emotional problem she had had for years. Another gained a closer relationship with God. Not everyone has these. What I found on my twenty-day cleanse was that the second ten days for me were learning to handle problems without turning to food. In addition to that valuable lesson, I also gained a much more pleasant and even-tempered disposition. I think that these benefits are perhaps the reasons many religions and Indian tribes use fasts to help the spiritual nature of man.

Emotional eating

One benefit I gained from my twenty-day cleanse was the ability to face stress without handling it with food.

I have braved through the Master Cleanse 3 times now. I'm not going to lie, it can be a tough experience and put you face to face with personal challenges like what role does food play in your life? Food satisfied me on many levels other than just something in my stomach. I realized I ate for many reasons... boredom, anxiety, thirst, etc. The MC made me face these challenges which made me feel a lot freer in the end, because I no longer used food as a crutch but rather one of the multiple means to good health. ... Here's to Better Health! Your body will thank you…

M.
September 25, 2007

Exercise, running, and weights

There are two types of exercise: Those that strengthen the heart and circulation (aerobic) and those that build muscle. Running, jogging, and bicycling are examples of aerobic exercise. This type of exercise is very compatible with the Master Cleanse. In fact, most people report being able to do better for longer periods while on the MC, with the occasional detox day—usually Days 2, 3, 7, 14—where you may feel tired. But in general most people have much more energy. Muscle building, however, is not compatible with the Master Cleanse as there is no protein with which to rebuild muscles. Just in case you are worried about going without protein for ten, twenty or more days, Joel Fuhrman, MD, makes the point in his book, *Fasting—and Eating—for Health,* that the average non-overweight person has enough nutrient reserves to fast for at least forty days.

My first MC fast was for 38 days. I have seen several questions about exercise during the fast. In my own experience I felt that exercise was a very good idea as I believe it helps the body cleanse better than not exercising. I rode my bike about 35 miles every other day. I just could not believe the energy I had.

I took the lemon mixture with me in my water bottles, which kept my blood sugar up and fueled my body. In 38 days I lost a whopping 36 pounds! I think it very important for people to know this cleanse is about detox, not weight loss, although I found that my body has remained 20 pounds lighter to this day. So I gained back about half the weight I lost. I started at 213 pounds and went all the way to 175. I got a little concerned and [it was] the main reason I broke the fast.

Orange Juice never tasted so good... I have since done the fast twice. [A] little over a year has passed from the first fast; a 10-day with no weight loss at all and a 15-day where I lost 15 pounds. It seems the amount of exercise I do on the fast has, of course, a direct effect on the amount of weight loss and I assume the amount of undesirable waste products I eliminate. Keeping good circulation going in the body makes a great deal of sense to me.

G.
March 8, 2004

Friends and family

Don't announce the cleanse to every person you meet. Don't argue with the uneducated. Don't try to convince other people. Don't set yourself up for failure or negative feedback. Tell those close friends who you know will support you on your great adventure.

Hair loss

Very rarely (perhaps 1 out of 500 or so), a woman (I have never heard it happening to a man) temporarily loses more hair than usual after a cleanse. In every case, their hair has grown back. In the two cases I checked into personally, both women had done cleanses once a month for at least three months in a row. In each case taking extra vitamins, minerals and healthy food produced new, healthy hair. I have heard it said that it results from lack of protein, but this doesn't make sense as what about the other 499 who went without protein for as many or more days. I believe it may result from a lack of alkaline mineral reserves (calcium, magnesium, potassium and sodium) due to too many cleanses too close together. The toxins that are being detoxified are acids and need to be neutralized by the alkaline minerals mentioned above. This is why I recommend waiting at least three months between cleanses. Strangely, I have never heard of anyone losing hair regardless of how long their cleanse went. I have heard from people who have gone forty and even sixty-eight days. It only seems to occur if a person does monthly Master Cleanses for at least three months in a row.

Headaches on first days

Coming off a heavy caffeine habit (coffee, sodas, or tea) on the cleanse occasionally causes headaches even in people who eat healthy food and are otherwise in good shape. If you are coming off caffeine, be sure to have six to twelve drinks of the lemonade each day along with plenty of water to wash out the toxins. In addition, be sure to follow the instructions on the salt water flush and the laxative tea. You want to eliminate as many of the toxins as fast as you can. Most important of all, recognize that the headaches are detox symptoms from quitting a caffeine addiction. They usually go away in one or two days. The most I have heard of are four days. Persist.

I just finished my first 10 day MC on Tuesday. I am now Day 3 post cleanse and am completely caffeine FREE!! I've been a morning coffee drinker for the past 22 yrs and this is the longest I've EVER gone without coffee and I feel great!

Yes, I had a 10-hour headache from HELL on Day 1, it's true. I suffered in excruciating pain and threw up three times during those ten hours, but I knew it would pass and my body was releasing what it didn't need, so I hung in there and didn't give in to the temptation to take [a pain medication], either. I used lavender essential oil on my temples to help with the pain. It helped a lot.

Since that first day, I've had no headaches and have continued to wake up each morning feeling energized and refreshed. I'm now drinking hot lemon water in the mornings and plan to continue for as long as I can.

By not giving yourself the chance to break this habit, you don't get to experience the self-empowerment that comes from conquering your addiction. You are MUCH stronger than you give yourself credit for. Take it from one who knows....a true caffeine addict.

Shine
Central Coast, CA
April 28, 2006

Health—attitudes about

1. Each person is responsible for her or his own health.

2. It is wise for a person to learn how to maintain and/or improve their health.

3. Valuable knowledge is available if you take the time to look for it and are willing to determine for yourself whether any knowledge presented is true or false.

4. Each person's body is potentially different. For example, most people find penicillin valuable for killing bacteria. Some people are allergic and might die from it.

5. Diagnosis or advice from a health professional is frequently essential, but each person is responsible to determine if it is true or not for his or her own body and whether to follow the treatment.

6. You must use your own good judgment and experience if you decide to apply the knowledge in my book or on my website or forum. Do not accept it blindly. This may mean consulting a licensed healthcare practitioner.

Hemorrhoids

A friend had a history of hemorrhoids. On the second day of the cleanse he got bleeding hemorrhoids, but they were not as painful as before. A few days later they went away. He feels they will never come back as long as he keeps his diet relatively clean.

High blood pressure

Fasting is known to reduce high blood pressure. In fact, there is a scientific study done on 174 people with high blood pressure. After a ten-day water fast, everyone on medication was able to come off it. In Germany, Japan and Russia, there are annual medical conferences on the benefits of fasting. The 2000 Russian conference heard papers citing the benefits of fasting for treating ten different diseases including asthma, bronchitis, hypertension (high blood pressure), viral lung infections and obesity.

This book makes a lot of claims such as the various symptoms that can be remedied by doing the Master Cleanse. I was a GREAT BIG SKEPTIC. As a person who suffers with asthma, allergies, inflammation, sinus congestion, high blood pressure (HBP), and leg edema, I have been on medications from my doctors for many years. I found it hard to believe the words and claims of those in the book. However, I have done the Master Cleanse (Lemonade Diet) and all I can say is BELIEVE THE HYPE!! It WORKS! After 15 days, my edema had lessened greatly, my sinus congestion had disappeared as did my chest congestion. I haven't had to take my High blood pressure medication and I test my HBP daily because I found this outcome the hardest to believe. I had been told I'd be on my HBP medicine for life. Best of all, I feel better, my thinking is clearer and I have more energy. I still have some allergies and inflammation blockages but I am going to do the Master Cleanse every season. However first, I plan to go back on the cleanse again in the next month. This time, I want to stay on it until my currently coated tongue becomes a healthy pink – the true sign of health. Oh, by the way, I lost 10 lbs. but although I need to lose more, I was more interested in the other health benefits that I received as a result. Buy this book and go on the cleanse—you won't be sorry. The cleanse ingredients are cheaper than most medications and it is better for you because everything is natural. If you care about yourself, do this for yourself.

R. Pryor
New York
June 17, 2007

Honey

Burroughs says never use honey internally. It is predigested by bees and goes directly into the blood stream—like alcohol—spiking blood sugar and prompting the body to reduce it by secreting insulin, which lowers the blood sugar, but promotes depression. I don't go so far as to say never to use honey internally. However, I don't use or recommend people substituting honey for maple syrup for the Master Cleanse. The maple syrup provides many alkaline minerals, including sodium, potassium, calcium, and magnesium, necessary to neutralize acidic toxins. I was once contacted by a man in India who couldn't find maple syrup, so he used honey. After the cleanse, he said his teeth became loose. Don't use honey for the Master Cleanse. If you cannot find maple syrup, use fresh sugar cane juice.

Hunger vs. cravings

Frequently, people confuse hunger with cravings. The way to distinguish between hunger and cravings is to ask yourself if you are interested in eating an apple, some carrots or a fresh green salad. If you are interested in those, you are hungry. If they are not appealing, but you are interested in ribs, French fries, a hamburger, etc., you are experiencing cravings. As cravings are a detox symptom, they will reduce or disappear with your next morning's eliminations if you are doing the Master Cleanse as written.

True hunger occurs in only about one quarter of the people doing the Master Cleanse. The rest feel no hunger at all no matter how long they cleanse. This is similar to people who do water fasts. Hunger disappears after Day 2 and doesn't reappear until the fast is complete. (This was one of my findings from a survey or 141 people who had done the Master Cleanse at one time or another.) It is possible these hungry people simply didn't drink enough lemonade or water. I have read that a single glass of water will turn off hunger in more than 90% of people on diets. Two people who experienced hunger, not cravings, that I talked to personally both had taken diet pills for some years. So it might have been due to detoxification of the diet pills. So I now know of four possibilities for hunger: 1) The person is not drinking another glass of lemonade or water, 2) The person is eating or drinking something in addition to the lemonade, salt water, or tea and that is creating or perpetuating the hunger; 3) The person is perceiving cravings as hunger; or 4) The person has a history of diet pills.

Lost 29 lbs in 14 days in March 07. I'm a big guy and normally eat more than 4000 calories per day. So I thought I would be really hungry but surprisingly I wasn't. Certainly there were times when I was but overall it wasn't that hard. You find out how much of your eating is habit or boredom and not really caused by hunger. My energy levels were also high, in fact some nights I had trouble sleeping.

J.B.
Provo, Utah
September 25, 2007

Hypoglycemia/low blood sugar

People with hypoglycemia, or low blood sugar, are sometimes concerned because they have been told they have to eat every few hours. This is not a problem on the Master Cleanse provided you drink enough lemonade drinks to keep your blood sugar up in the first few days. After that, fasting (and the Master Cleanse is a juice fast) is known to normalize blood sugar so it will not be a problem later in the cleanse.

Infertility and the cleanse

There are numerous mentions of infertility being handled by fasting. One for example is explained in the chapter, "Sterility In Women," in *Fasting Can Save Your Life* by Herbert M. Shelton. Shelton, a naturopath or doctor of naturopathy, fasted between 30,000 and 40,000 patients to health, including Joel Fuhrman, MD, author of *Eat to Live*, who was inspired to become a doctor by this experience. Shelton tells of many cases where women, previously infertile and unable to conceive, conceived and delivered healthy children within a few weeks or months of fasting. I am aware of two women who were unable to conceive who did so within a few months of completing the Master Cleanse.

Interrupting the cleanse

People have asked if they could "break" the cleanse with orange juice and/or grapefruit juice for a few days and then get back on it without losing the weight loss and cleansing benefits. I do not recommend it. Just orange juice or grapefruit juice might be okay for one day, but it will not sustain you for many days in a row.

Intestinal/abdominal cramps

Due to less waste in the intestines, you can sometimes feel intestinal contractions. Occasionally, they are uncomfortable. This can be handled by drinking more lemonade or water to give the intestines something to push. This generally handles it within a few minutes. Long term, use an herbal tea that is a combination of herbs rather than pure senna leaf or only drink half of the cup of laxative tea.

Laxative tea

Laxative dependency

I have never heard of anyone who has become dependent on either the salt water flush or the laxative tea from doing the Master Cleanse. I've read the warnings on the laxative tea boxes, but in the more than 2,000 cleanses I know about, not one person ever became dependent on the laxative tea.

Laxative tea

No special laxative tea is recommended by Burroughs. He never specifies "senna." He only says herbal laxative tea. I recommend a tea with about 50% senna leaf. You can find them at your local health food store. Straight senna can be too powerful when there is not much in the colon to expel. Use a senna blend (50% senna and 50% other herbs) or only drink half of the cup you made. On the other hand, if you are not eliminating much of anything, you might want to try pure senna tea for a few days. Drink it only the last thing at night just before you go to sleep. It should take six to twelve hours before it causes eliminations. Sometimes it is faster. That way your eliminations will be right when you wake up in the morning instead of in the middle of the night.

Lemonade and lemons

Bottled or frozen lemon juice

Bottled juice is a no-no as the vitamins and enzymes that do the good work are destroyed by time, sunlight and cooking (pasteurizing). Even if you find non-pasteurized "raw" or frozen lemon juice, after several hours most of the enzymes are destroyed by time. Concerning the high prices of organic ingredients for the cleanse, my wife and I figured that its about $16.75 per day including the cost of maple syrup, lemons, sea salt and laxative tea. Although not required, it is well worth it. When you finish the cleanse, you will discover that you don't eat as much any more, so rather than eat foods that have had all their enzymes and vitamins removed and then had preservatives and pesticides added, why not spend the same money for fewer high-quality (organic) foods with real nutrition? One of the things I have learned from my research into nutrition and healing is that proper nutrition equals a pleasant, serene attitude toward life. The spiritual side starts to show through.

Including the lemon skin and pulp

Blending some of the skin (organic lemons only) and pulp can enhance the work of the lemon during your period to prevent clotting internally. (It doesn't, however, interfere with normal menstrual periods.) You must peel the rind on non-organic ones. Then put the whole thing through the juicer.

Juicing lemons

I have done it two ways: using an expensive juicer with whole organic lemons and with just squeezing the lemons. The taste is quite different, but I got the same results both ways. It is not required to use organic lemons or limes. If you are only squeezing them and not putting them through a juicer, you needn't peel the rind on non-organic ones. That is only if you are going to put the whole thing through the juicer.

More or less lemon juice?

Burroughs says to never to vary the amount of lemon juice in each drink. You can increase or decrease the maple syrup, but not the amount of the lemon juice.

Not drinking enough lemonade

If you don't drink the minimum, you won't detoxify as much or as fast. Lots of fluids help cleanse the kidneys and liver as well as the colon. One way to get down more lemonade is to drink only lemonade until you reach your minimum of six drinks. Drink your first glass about one-half to one hour after the salt water. Then drink a glass every hour. This will make you pee frequently. Every time you pee, drink another glass.

Premixing the lemonade

Let's face it. You have to premix enough to last through the day if you are going to go to work outside your house. However, I have heard of people squeezing lemons and mixing the maple syrup as a "premix" that they then add to water over the next two or more days. (Never use commercial bottled juice! It is pasteurized and old = no enzymes.) If you have read anything about the wheatgrass diet, the Hippocrates diet, the raw food diet, the Gerson anti-degenerative disease regimen, juicing for health or the Optimum Health Institute, you know that enzymes diminish over time, even in as little time as a few hours. You cannot get away from having to make enough to get through the day, but making more than one day's supply (even a day and an evening) will diminish your benefits. Also, if you do make a premix daily, do not add the cayenne until you are ready to drink. Cayenne will get hotter as it sits in liquid.

> Best detox plan — I did the Master Cleanse once and what a difference for me. I am a truck driver and am always eating fast food on the road. I had gained a lot of weight and had headaches all the time. I started the cleanse making 3 32 oz. bottles of the lemonade to drink each day. Not one time during the cleanse did I have any hunger pangs or feel weak from not eating... My headaches went away and I felt great. The hardest part was mentally stopping myself from eating, out of boredom, not from hunger. I am now starting the cleanse again... this time longer. Thanks....
>
> D. W.
> Michigan
> August 13, 2007

When to drink the lemonade

When you mix up a pitcher of the lemonade, you can drink the lemonade whenever you want. I would wait at least a half hour to one hour after the salt water. Finish drinking it at least two hours before going to sleep. Then you don't have to wake up to use the bathroom. Drink the laxative tea just before you go to sleep. These are not Master Cleanse instructions, just my suggestions.

Lemons—how many do I buy?

A large lemon will yield two ounces of juice. So, for six drinks a day, you will need three large lemons per day or thirty for ten days. If you buy organic lemons, only get enough for 5 days as that is the longest they last in the refrigerator. Limes are great for a change of pace. They are smaller and you will need about twice as many of them to make a drink. Burroughs says you can use either lemons or limes. I prefer the taste of lemons for the long run, but occasional drinks with lime are kind of fun.

Madal Bal syrup/Neera cleanse

Here is what I know about Madal Bal syrup and the Neera Super Cleanse. In 2004, I recall they advertised Madal Bal syrup as a refinement by Stanley Burroughs himself and it was still called the Master Cleanse. Now it is called the Neera Super Cleanse and the story is that others in Europe researched a better syrup. The location of Europe is important. There is no maple syrup produced in Europe. So, the importing of maple syrup from the US or Canada would be very expensive. This may account for the use of an alternative in Europe. Furthermore, they claim that it includes Grade C maple syrup which is a grade no longer used by the US Dept of Agriculture, which regulates the US grades, and Canada uses a numbered system. Regardless of the above facts, it is much more expensive than maple syrup in the US and it is a questionable replacement. In countries where freshly extracted sugar cane juice is available, Burroughs says that is ideal. I personally stick with organic Grade B maple syrup, although I would love to try the freshly extracted sugar cane juice version if I could find it.

Maple syrup cravings

If you have a craving for additional maple syrup, try increasing the amount in the drink to the full two tablespoons rather than eating the maple syrup separately. This will keep your blood sugar level more constant and reduce your craving for an extra teaspoon of maple syrup now and then.

Medication

Blood thinners, Coumadin

Be advised that the Master Cleanse will thin the blood. So, if you are on blood-thinning medication, you will need to work with your licensed healthcare practitioner to adjust dosages. I spoke to a man recently who loved what the Master Cleanse did for him, but he was pulled off it twice by his doctor who had him on a blood thinner and his tests showed it was too thin each time on the Master Cleanse. That doctor refused to adjust his dosage. So, he found another doctor willing to adjust it while he was on the Master Cleanse.

High blood pressure

Be sure to run the concept of the cleanse lowering blood pressure by your doctor for coordination purposes to make sure you don't get a double whammy from the combined effects of the medication and the cleanse and faint when you stand up. Fasting is known to reduce high blood pressure. In fact, there is a scientific study done on 174 people with high blood pressure. After a ten-day water fast, everyone on medication was able to come off it. Be sure you stand or sit up slowly.

Prescription meds

I am not a medical doctor and even if I were, I don't have your complete medical history, chart and any diagnostic test results. So, I would not even dream of advising you as to whether you should discontinue your medicine. You should seek the advice of your licensed healthcare provider and use your own good judgment. Here is some information that you may find useful to help make your decision.

1. The purpose of a cleanse is to remove toxins and old waste from the body. The body in most cases treats medical drugs as toxins from a digestive standpoint. So, putting more in while trying to get toxins out doesn't make a lot of sense. Thus, you may consider eliminating any NON-PRESCRIBED medicines, such as allergy, diet or sleeping pills that were not prescribed by a licensed healthcare professional. If you are on a prescribed medication,

especially such as that to avoid a heart attack, stroke or other fatal event, do NOT discontinue your medicine without consulting a licensed healthcare practitioner!

2. In some cases, the body stores some of the medicine it is taking in the fat cells. Max Gerson, MD (www.gerson.org), reported that anywhere between 20%–40% of each dose of chemotherapy medicine is stored in the body and could be released during detoxification. I believe this is likely with strong psychiatric medicines also. I recommend people who have been on chemotherapy or strong psychiatric medicines within the last six months do a much gentler and slower detox. You can always come back to the Master Cleanse later after you have done a slower form of detox.

3. As far as doing the cleanse while being on the medication, in a January 2005 survey of 141 people who have done or were doing the Master Cleanse, only one person reported having any problems at all with her medication. And that lady only had a problem once, but went on and did the cleanse nine more times!

Mucoid plaque

Mucoid plaque is a tough rubbery coating that forms from mucus and accumulated waste on the large intestine walls. There are numerous pictures of this on the Web. I have only heard of one person who described an elimination that could have been mucoid plaque. Most of the time, the accumulated waste is just dissolved over several days by the lemon juice and cayenne, washed by the salt water, and broken up into small mucousy flakes by the increased intestinal action brought on by the herbal laxative tea. That is always been the case for me. I think anyone wanting to see foot-long sections (or longer) of mucoid plaque needs to do a colon cleanse with psyllium and/or bentonite clay that mechanically pushes the waste out rather than the Master Cleanse. Personally, I prefer the Master Cleanse.

Nothing happening on MC

Let's look at all the points where this cleanse could go wrong and see if we can sort it out.

1. Are you putting two teaspoons of non-iodized sea salt in the salt water each morning and drinking it as fast as possible?

2. Are you mixing two tablespoons (one ounce) of fresh squeezed—not bottled—lemon juice into each ten-ounce drink or using these proportions for each batch and making no more than one day's worth at a time?

3. Are you putting in at least 1/10 teaspoon of cayenne pepper or less and gradually increasing the amount to taste with each drink?

4. Are you drinking one cup of laxative tea each morning as well as each evening to encourage more elimination?

5. Are you eating or drinking anything else but water and occasional mint tea?

6. Before this cleanse, did you have only one or two BMs per week? Being constipated before the cleanse might mean a little longer before you would see results.

7. Are you on any constipating medications? I am NOT suggesting you come off any prescribed medications. Just that they may alter the results of the cleanse. The only other thought I have for anyone not seeing results by Day 5 is that some people who have lived on the SAD diet (Standard American Diet) and are overweight may take a while before enough accumulated waste is loosened and eliminated to start seeing results. Go for the full ten days. That is what Burroughs says. Big changes usually come after Day 7. Yes, some people get results more quickly than others, but do not judge your results by what happens after five, six or seven days. My wife learned that there were many days when she did not lose pounds, but then she discovered that she was losing inches. Her body was changing shape for the better rather than losing weight. Take a longer view. If you get enough lemonade and cayenne, you will not be straining to try to make it to Day 6. You will be cruising with the rest of us.

● Osteoporosis

Overeating meat, fat, sugar and processed foods produces an acid condition in the body. This is added to by artificial sweeteners, colors, preservatives and flavors as well as medicines, all of which are treated by the body as acidic toxins. In order to neutralize these, the liver must have alkaline minerals (calcium, magnesium, potassium and sodium). If it doesn't have enough reserves, it must take them from the bones and teeth as the blood must be slightly alkaline. Osteoporosis is the result of taking calcium from the bones. Dental cavities are the result of taking them from the teeth. The current abundance of osteoporosis and concern about calcium is the result of not eating an 80% alkaline diet, that is to say, not enough green salads and raw fruits and vegetables.

Other cleanses—Liver/kidney/parasite cleanse

Stanley Burroughs, the developer of the Master Cleanse, says it will cleanse all the organs, glands and joints, including the kidneys and liver. People with arthritis have even commented that they noticed joint pain relieved or eliminated. From experience, I know that the Master Cleanse handles many parasites because I have noticed when I pick my nose before a cleanse, I don't afterward. (That is one of the symptoms of parasites. Some of the others being itchy anus, fatigue and overeating.) Other nutritional, natural healers, including Norman Walker, have said parasites require waste accumulations in order to find good breeding grounds. So it makes sense that the Master Cleanse also handles many parasites.

Changed my life the first cleanse. I am on day 13 of the Master Cleanse. I have been off all my medications. I have had no pain from my rheumatoid arthritis. Four weeks ago I was walking with a cane. I have not had an asthma attack, my thyroid has not given me any trouble. I look younger and feel younger, my skin is baby soft. I have more energy than I thought possible. Thank you Peter you gave me my life back.

M.H.
September 25, 2007

DYNAMITE!!!!!!!!!!!!!!!! I lost 17 1/2 pounds in 17 days, also lost liver spots & skin tags and my skin cleared up—I look 10 years younger according to all the compliments received!!!!!!! Oh yeah—hip pain GONE and my eye sight is clearer also! The list of improvements goes on and on…. Felt GREAT with lots of energy and YES I did detox boy did I de-tox—best cleanse ever—did my cleanse in February of 07 and planning on one for May!

K.W.
March 26, 2007

I'm going for 20 days! My response to the Master Cleanse so far is: I am amazed at the energy level I have. I feel better now than when I am eating food. To be able to get up every morning at 5:00 AM, do my 8-hour a day, stressful job, come home and still be up and moving around is incredible! Aches & pains (arthritis) have vanished. Sleep is much improved. I crave quiet now. I always used to go to bed with the TV on. Now I want QUIET. I am calmer now and would much rather read to relax, then fall asleep. No more annoying TV noise is needed or wanted…. I now feel like I have discovered the "Fountain of Youth!" This cleanse is do-able, and it definitely works. I have lost some weight and am feeling so good…. Y'all [Peter and Marlene] are great motivators. So please keep up the good work!

S.I.
Lakeland, FL
June 2004

Parasites—Will the cleanse get rid of parasites?

This cleanse definitely gets rid of many kinds. I have read that one of the signs of parasites is picking the nose (yes, it is that common). After about five days on the cleanse, my nose picking stopped. It doesn't come back as long as I don't eat meat. Once I start on ribs (my favorite) or other types of meat, I start again. The parasites need accumulated acid waste matter to survive. A clean, healthy bowel will not support them. This is just another bonus of the Master Cleanse.

● Passing gas—Warning

I am sorry, but there is no delicate way to say this and IT MUST BE SAID: After you have done the salt water flush for the first time UNTIL YOU COMPLETE THE MASTER CLEANSE, if you feel the need to fart or pass gas, be sure you are on the toilet first. A lot of funny stories result from not following this advice.

Protein

Do vegetarians get protein?

The average person needs 30–50 grams of protein a day. That is 1–1.5 ounces per day! In addition, T. Colin Campbell, Ph.D., nutritional researcher and author of *The China Study*, points out that although meat contains all the essential proteins we need to build our bodies, plants also contain these proteins and by eating an assortment of vegetables we easily meet our protein requirement with proteins that are healthier for us. In *The Wheatgrass Book* by Ann Wigmore, she talks about a raw fruit/vegetable/nut/seed diet along with wheatgrass juice as supplying all the needed protein and other nutrients to rebuild the body.

Remember, the largest land animals are vegetarians. They have no trouble building huge muscular bodies with protein. If you feel you need more protein, start adding soaked almonds and seeds to your diet as well. (Soaking the almonds releases the enzyme inhibiter—the substance that keeps them from sprouting—and makes them easier to digest.) For example, spirulina has more than 60% protein by weight compared to beef or chicken, which have about 20%, which is about the same as sunflower seeds and almonds. Eggs have less than 5%, about the same as broccoli and cauliflower. (SOURCE: Paul Pitchford, *Healing with Whole Foods*, p.143)

Will I get enough protein?

Joel Fuhrman, MD, makes the point in his book *Fasting and Eating for Health* that the average non-overweight person has enough nutrient reserves to fast for at least forty days.

Quitting on detox days

In general, don't end your cleanse on a detox day. The Master Cleanse is a rapid form of detoxification so it will usually handle the detox symptoms much faster than if you are eating normally. The exception to that is if you have a detox symptom that hasn't gone away in a few days. If you are experiencing severe detox symptoms and they are not going away after a few days, it may be better to go off the cleanse and slow down the detoxification.

Salt water flush

How to do the salt water flush

Put two level TEASPOONS of non-iodized sea salt in thirty-two ounces of water. Non-iodized means no iodine has been added. Sea salt will already contain iodine naturally, but none has been added to that. Drink that as quickly as you can. The water may be warm or cold as you wish. The reason for the salt is to make the relative weight of the water (scientifically known as the specific gravity) match that of blood so that the kidneys don't absorb the water and the blood doesn't absorb the salt. Then all of it can wash through the system in a very dramatic way.

Importance of the salt water flush

It is important to understand that there are two parts to this cleanse. Part one is the detox: mobilizing the waste from the parts of the body where it is stored. This is accomplished by not eating. Part two is elimination: ensuring the waste is washed out of the body quickly and regularly so that the toxins are not reabsorbed, which will make you feel sick or miserable. Part two is composed of two parts. The "Agitator" is the laxative tea, which stimulates the muscles of the intestines to contract and push the waste along. And "The Rinse Cycle" is the salt water flush. It was Stanley Burroughs' genius to add these elimination actions to make detox symptoms less or eliminate them entirely.

Nothing happening on the salt water flush

Some people find that drinking the salt water doesn't produce any eliminations for the first couple days. Usually this is true of those who eat meat or dairy products regularly. Adjusting the salt (usually increasing it) does the trick. If you haven't gotten the salt water flush to work by Day 3, switch to another cup of laxative tea in the morning, and try the salt water flush again around Day 8.

Sea salt for the salt water flush

Follow Burroughs' instructions on using sea salt and not table salt. I have heard from a few people who tried using table salt and they told me the taste is very much worse than sea salt. The term sea salt can include those salts that are mined from prehistoric salt beds.

Salt water flush troubles

Some people gag on the taste. It is much easier to take if you use the non-iodized sea salt that Burroughs says to use. My wife recommends using a straw so that the taste isn't so strong or counting the number of swallows to take your mind off the taste. I have never had a problem. I have found that the salt water flush is easier to do as I go through the cleanse and have less waste in my intestines. Later days are easier than earlier days and later cleanses are easier than early cleanses.

If you cannot tolerate the salt water flush, drink another cup of laxative tea in the morning as well as the one at night. Be sure you are using non-iodized sea salt. You could also try to drink it with a straw really quickly so you don't have to taste it.

Salt water flush warnings

The salt water flush should be done only when nothing else has been eaten or drunk before it that day. I learned this the hard way and know of one other person who has done the salt water flush in the middle of the day after lemonade and was quite nauseated.

Also, don't add anything to flavor the water. One person added soy sauce. That is a mistake because soy sauce contains protein, which requires significant digestive work. It is like drinking steak or cooked meat as far as the digestive process is concerned.

What to expect on the salt water flush

Within thirty to sixty minutes after drinking the salt water most people have several urgent, intense eliminations. These generally last for the next 30 to 60 minutes. So, be sure you are close to a bathroom you don't have to wait for during this time. If you are planning on leaving your house, give yourself two hours from the time you drink it until you have to leave the house. If you have had any detox symptoms the previous day, you can expect them to be gone or reduced after these eliminations.

IT'S A GREAT FEELING. Wanted to let everyone know that I have finished the fast that was started on Jan. 2, 2008 and finished on Jan. 31, 2008 (30 days). I am very overweight and did not weigh myself before I started however, I believe you really don't have to because you can tell just by how you feel, the way your clothes fit and the energy you start to get after the initial phase. In March I plan on doing it again for the ten days only, till I totally clean myself out.

My problems with the salt water solution I solved by using the SENNA tea from the health food store once at night before I went to bed and once at work in the morning and it worked great for me. It did its job. Along with the fast I have now started to try and (mostly) be a vegetarian with poultry and fish somewhat and meat on rare occasions. So far so good on that venture with vegetable soup almost every day with fruits and seeds / nuts and organic wheat breads, pasta etc. when I can.

E.
February 11, 2008

Shopping List

The only variable is the number of ten-ounce drinks you will have per day. It should be between six and twelve. I have used six in the estimate below.

1. 6 gallons of spring, distilled or purified water without chlorine and not fluoridated. (This amount includes the salt water flush.)

2. 30 large lemons or 60 limes or a combination (organic preferred, but not required)

3. 60 fl. oz. organic Grade B maple syrup

4. 1/4 pound non-iodized sea salt (I recommend Light Grey Celtic Sea Salt.)

5. 1/4 ounce of cayenne pepper

6. ten herbal laxative tea servings in bags

7. herbal mint tea (optional)

All of these things are readily available at most health food stores or can be conveniently ordered from www.TheMasterCleanse.com/store.

Skin

Clear skin

Clear skin is an indicator that you are no longer overloading your digestive system with toxins that have to be eliminated. One of the organs of elimination is the skin. When you cease putting cooked food, meat, dairy, artificial colors, flavors and preservatives into your body, your skin clears up quickly as it no longer needs to eliminate "junk," which is what makes your skin look old and ill.

It really works!!!! In 2005, I began gaining weight in spite of the fact that I was eating healthy and exercising regularly. I became very discouraged, especially since I could not pinpoint a cause for the sudden weight gain. I had my thyroid tested and underwent other tests as well. According to the tests, all was well. I was relieved, but still perplexed. Then, one day I heard about the Master Cleanse. I researched the cleanse and its simplicity intrigued me. I was uncertain whether I'd be able to drink the "lemonade" concoction for 10 days, but I was willing to try. ... During the cleanse, my night sweats ceased, my acne cleared up and my allergy symptoms went away. I was so excited about the results I achieved after 10 days that I went six extra days. As a result, I have lost over 20 lbs. and kept it off. My body simply craved better foods after the cleanse and I didn't argue with it. I will probably do this cleanse quarterly for the rest of my life and recommend it to anyone "willing" to try it.

T.D.
New Jersey
January 10, 2007

Skin rash

A rash is a detox symptom. If it is moving around, it shows that change is happening. Detoxing is a change. We want that. A detox day (rash, drainage, etc.) is not a day to stop. You will be happy afterward.

Smoking & the cleanse

Will smoking prevent you from getting the benefits of the Master Cleanse? Like the rest of life, it is relative. If you are a smoker and you continue to smoke on the cleanse, your benefits will be less than if you were not smoking. How much less? I do not know. I have heard from smokers that they have gotten good results. If you do want to quit, you will find that it is much easier to quit as the toxins creating the cravings will be speedily eliminated and thus lessen your desires. This may also be true for alcoholics and drug addicts. Burroughs does say it is the case.

The Cleanse helped me break my food and alcohol addiction by realizing I don't need anything to change my mood, I can be pure and happy.

D.C.
Florida
March 26, 2007

Stop smoking with the master cleanse. I am getting ready to start my second Master cleanse in a few weeks. My first time was about six months ago. I was joined by my sister, her boyfriend and my sister in law. We were all successful in our own way. My sister and her boyfriend quit smoking cold turkey on day one and have not gone back. They both would agree this was the easiest way to quit with the least amount of negative side effects. I am excited about doing the cleanse again.

E.Z.
September 28, 2007

I just wanted to thank you. I am on day 7 of the MC and I feel great. I donated a kidney years ago and never stopped taking the pain meds. I had tried several times to quit, but it never worked. I stopped using opiates the same day I started the MC.

I really believe that the strict rules of the cleanse, the true desire to finally be healthy and the ease of the MC have helped. I have huge headaches, but that could very well be withdrawal from the opiates as opposed to the MC. I am working out every day. [The Master Cleanse] has changed my life!

A.
July 14, 2010

Spiritual experience

Fasting has been used for thousands of years to produce a temporary heightening of spiritual experience. This is not true for everyone who does the Master Cleanse, but it has happened to some. Here is a quote from one of them.

Anyone besides myself have any spiritual encounters?? I had mine on Day 5. I felt Him deep, a feeling so unexplainable that I have never had before. I had uncontrollable streaming tears practically on my knees (weeping), along with some very, very strange coincidences and I don't believe in coincidences. I've always been a believer. I am now convinced about my beliefs and I am in complete bliss!

My first motive for this cleanse was weight loss; it has now changed to a spiritual motive. Let my new journey begin!

A.

Starvation—Isn't this starving yourself?

The only similarity is that both involve no feeding. In his million-copy bestseller, *Fasting, The Ultimate Diet*, Allan Cott, MD has 329 citations supporting fasting. 158 are scientific journal articles. He even includes a quotation from *The New England Journal of Medicine*: "Fasting is a valid experience. It can benefit any otherwise healthy person whose calories now have the upper hand in his/her life." In Germany, Japan and Russia, there are annual medical conferences on the benefits of fasting. The 2000 Russian conference heard papers citing the benefits of fasting for treating ten different diseases including asthma, bronchitis, hypertension (high blood pressure), viral lung infections and obesity. The Russian doctor, Yuri Nikolayev, of the Moscow Psychiatric Research Institute was famous for treating 7,000 mental patients successfully with fasting alone after other forms of treatment failed!

Substitutes for maple syrup

Fresh sugar cane juice (notice, that is not cane syrup) is better than maple syrup and sorghum is worse than maple syrup. Diabetics should use molasses at first, then switch to maple syrup.

Surgery and the MC

Ask your surgeon by what date he expects you to be healed completely. Then there will be no question about whether you are getting enough protein to heal the operation scar while you are on the cleanse.

Teas on the MC

Occasional mint tea and herbal laxative tea in the evening and optionally in the morning are the only teas Burroughs lists in his book.

Time between cleanses—How soon can I do it again?

How soon can you do another Master Cleanse? It is best to space out your Master Cleanses by three or four months and eat lots of fresh greens and salads in between or drink daily green smoothies. You need to build up your calcium, magnesium and potassium reserves because that is what the body uses to neutralize the toxins before they are eliminated. Very rarely (three out of a thousand), a person has done a Master Cleanse every month for several months in a row, which resulted in temporary hair loss. It was handled by taking lots of vitamins and minerals, but it is better to avoid that.

Tingling or pain in the teeth

A very small number of people develop sensitive teeth while on the cleanse. Others have concern about the lemon eating away at their enamel. This is a very rare problem, but for those who have experienced this, it is quite a serious concern. My wife had sensitive teeth on her cleanse and found that drinking lemonade through a straw helped, along with rinsing her mouth after each drink with water (not tap). I believe this ties in with people not having enough alkaline mineral reserves, as the teeth are one place the body can always go to get calcium to neutralize the acidic toxins. Anyone who has sensitive teeth for more than a day on the cleanse should try the straw and rinsing and if the teeth are still sensitive, they should discontinue the cleanse. Then, before doing another cleanse, they should be sure to have lots of greens either in salads and/or green smoothies. See *Green for Life*, Victoria Boutenko's book on green smoothies, for more information and some great recipes.

Tongue coating

Tongue color, shape and coating have been used for thousands of years in traditional Chinese medicine. It is quite amazing all the information that can be learned just from looking at the tongue! A white tongue indicates you are actually eliminating mucus in the intestines. This coating of the tongue is mentioned by nearly every fasting author. When the tongue becomes clean and pink again the cleanse is complete. Of course, you can stop the Master Cleanse any time you want, but after the tongue coating is gone you definitely should stop. You will discover that it gets very coated during the cleanse. I also had a furry tongue on the MC. I decided to continue the cleanse until my tongue was clear pink. It took twenty days. A friend did it and it took him twenty-six.

Weight loss

Keeping the weight off

I was 6′ 1″ and weighed a little over 230 pounds in June of 2002. I felt terrible, too. My wife had gone on a 100% raw vegetable and fruit diet about six months before this. After watching her getting healthier, younger looking and happier, I decided I wanted to feel that way too—even if it meant giving up foods I craved. So, I spent six months eating only raw food and dropped to 198 pounds eating as much raw fruit, vegetables, nuts and seeds as I wanted. Then on 4 Jan 2003, I started my first Master Cleanse. When I finished it on January 24, I weighed 175 pounds. Four years later, I was eating mostly raw, had done the cleanse several more times and weighed 175. So you can see that returning to a solid food diet is not necessarily going to make all the weight return. What you eat after you finish your cleanse determines whether you will keep off the weight, continue to lose or put it back on. The cleanse does make me and several others I have heard from want to eat healthier and does remove some cravings for those foods that are bad for your health. I don't feel that people have to give up the "bad" foods completely, just realize they are not daily nutrition, but fun. Keep their consumption in perspective.

The MASTER CLEANSE SAVED ME FROM A LIFE OF SEDENTARY OBESITY! Due to my inactivity and excessive calorie consumption (accidents which prevented me from exercising played a part), I became extremely sedentary. My once active metabolism had slowed to a snail's pace. I was tired all the time and, unfortunately, this led to more overeating. Taking in way more calories than I was expending, my body became accustomed to the "feedings" and I thought I was hungry even though I was way over my daily caloric intake. Also, when you overeat on a regular basis your stomach becomes stretches out and you cannot tell when you've had enough calories to sustain life… you're eating just to "eat," which isn't the purpose of eating at all. …

Fast forward to a few months ago. After doing five Master Cleanses (20 days, 10 days, 14 days, 32 days) I feel better and look better than I have in over 10 years. In addition to cleansing my body of all of the toxins built up in part from an extremely poor diet, the Master Cleanse enabled me to press "reboot" on my taste buds which set the stage for a clean and healthy food/mouth union. That was key to my success. I lost weight, which led to increased mobility, which led to being active again!

Thanks to the Master Cleanse I have shed all but 20 of the 80 pounds and kept them off. No more desire for pizza, cake, candy, etc. I CRAVE fresh fruits, veggies, and healthy foods. It's crazy but it's true! What we stuff our face with is approximately 80-95% responsible for our weight issues or lack thereof. Being active/fit assists in weight loss and health overall. It's really FOOD choices and the QUANTITY you eat, as well as "when" you consume the calories that is KEY KEY KEY KEY. I was surprised to find this out but SO glad I did before I was 100, 150, or 200 lbs overweight. The sooner you start, the better off you are. I recommend the Master Cleanse to everyone that can safely fast (consult your doctor). Once you do the cleanse and feel the difference, you'll no doubt do what I am doing (and thousands of others) and share your success with friends, family and anyone who will listen.

…You can't imaging how much easier it is to life live when you rid yourself of toxins which, if you're overweight, will help reset your eating habits. This combination will bring you to another level of health. As far as I'm concerned the benefits of the Master Cleanse far outweighs any sacrifice involved with fasting. Feeling better day in and day out is better than any food you could possibly put in your mouth. On that note, I'm off to the gym.

R.H.
August 18, 2008

Losing too much weight or being underweight?

When you stop eating, the liver has enough energy for twelve hours. After that, the body begins to break down muscle to produce needed energy. Two to three days later the body stops burning muscle mass and begins to burn fat, producing chemicals called ketones. Once fat is burned, muscle mass is preserved and the body begins to literally digest diseased cells, waste and fat. An extremely underweight friend of mine did the Master Cleanse for more than ten days. She only lost two pounds and those were lost right at the beginning. After the cleanse, she began to put on healthy weight. This same process is described in Allan Cott, MD's second book on fasting, *Fasting as a Way of Life*.

Losing weight after the MC

People lose down to their optimum weight (which is thin) while on a diet that is 100% raw veggies, fruit, nuts, seeds, sprouts, etc. Be sure to continue to drink plenty of water: one ounce of water for every two pounds of body weight and more if you are active. Also you need some sea salt each day as well. The cleanse alone won't necessarily make you lose every pound you wish to lose. It is just a good stepping stone. You must continue after the cleanse by eating more healthy and exercising regularly. There are no shortcuts. This is just a good way to get in the correct mindset for doing these things. The fact that you are eliminating, losing weight, and have energy shows that you are doing the cleanse correctly. Look at the bigger picture. It is doing a lot more for you than just weight loss. Keep in mind that excess weight is due to the excess fat that the body created to protect itself from the toxins. Once you have lost the toxins, the excess weight will melt off rapidly.

Not losing weight

My wife learned that there were many days when she did not lose pounds, but then she discovered that she was losing inches. Her body was changing shape for the better rather than losing weight. So, if you are not losing pounds, see if your clothes are fitting more loosely. You may be losing inches instead.

Why does detox = weight loss?

A diet high in meat, fat, sugar and processed foods (the Standard American Diet) will produce an acid condition in the body. In addition, the artificial sweeteners, colors, preservatives and flavors are treated by the body as toxins. What it cannot eliminate, it stores in fat cells. Lose the toxins...lose the fat! When you release the toxins with the cleanse or slower detoxification diet, such as eating only a raw vegetarian diet, the fat is no longer needed as the toxins are gone and the body sheds the fat.

Will I lose muscle?

When you stop eating, the liver has enough energy for twelve hours. After that, the body begins to break down muscle to produce needed energy. Two to three days later the body stops burning muscle mass and begins to burn fat, producing a chemical called ketones. Once fat is burned, muscle mass is preserved and the body begins to literally digest diseased cells, waste and fat. An extremely underweight friend of mine did the Master Cleanse for more than ten days. She only lost two pounds and those were lost right at the beginning. After the cleanse, she began to put on healthy weight. This same process is described in Allan Cott, MD's second book on fasting, *Fasting as a Way of Life*.

Women's issues

Birth control pills

I have received several questions about continuing birth control pills while on the Master Cleanse. I have now heard from several women that they have not had any problems, nor has anyone mentioned any problem.

Fibroid tumors

I was once giving a speech in a health food store and a woman in her mid-twenties came up and asked to speak to the group. She said she had never met me, but wanted to thank me because she had had fibroid tumors which disappeared during a Master Cleanse, which she started because she read my book. Alan Goldhamer, DC makes the point that proper fasting often dramatically reduces the size of fibroid tumors. J. Kunjufu, Ph.D. also points out that poor diet can lead to fibroid tumors. In addition to direct problems, such as heavy bleeding and tremendous pain, they can over time result in backache, kidney obstruction and even miscarriages. Among his recommendations to resolve or prevent these, he suggests fasting for one to three weeks; eating a vegetarian diet; drinking wheatgrass juice; exercise; daily enemas; herbs; removing cooked food, meat and dairy products from the diet; meditation and prayer.

Menstrual periods

Numerous women have reported that the Master Cleanse influences periods in several ways. Initially it may produce spotting or premature periods. This is because a woman's periods are a detoxification process. Occasionally it may bring on an extended period. Generally, by the end of the cleanse it tends to normalize periods and make them easier, the idea being that it is the toxins that make periods difficult.

Word of mouth

For half a century, the Master Cleanse has spread by word of mouth. Eight years of coaching more than 2,000 people has taught me that verbal instructions are like playing telephone, the game where each person whispers a message to the next person in line. The message received is NEVER the same as the original.

I want you and your friends to get the best possible results. That comes from doing exactly what Stanley Burroughs developed. Ensure they do by telling them to get *The Master Cleanser* by Burroughs, *Lose Weight, Have More Energy & Be Happier in 10 Days* by me, or this book so they have the correct instructions.

Afterword

IMAGINE POSSIBILITY WITHOUT LIMITS.

Possibility, you know, has a sensation.

Pure possibility, without limits, feels something like knowing for certain that you are about to achieve something you have dreamed of, and worked for, for years—only much more intense.

It feels like you're a star in the heavens radiating shining energy in all directions—above, below, forward, to the sides, behind—and you are sending this out—without limits, infinitely—throughout the universe to everyone and everything.

It is a feeling that is far too powerful to be contained in a body. It is much too large for it. It is too intense for it.

It is the greatest feeling imaginable...........and it is you.

Peter Glickman

17 February 2012

General Release and Waiver

THE UNDERSIGNED (HEREINAFTER I, ME OR MINE) UNDERSTANDS AND agrees that _____ (hereinafter Coach) is not a licensed health care practitioner in any state and does not diagnose, prescribe, treat or cure. I am consulting Coach solely for my own personal education. Anything I decide to do after speaking with Coach will be entirely my decision and no one else's. I am consulting with Coach solely as an individual and am not connected in any way with any local, state or federal government or professional organization.

I recognize that I am completely responsible for my own health and that it would be ludicrous to assume that anyone else can be responsible for my health. Even if I were to consult a licensed medical doctor, I would still be the final arbiter over whether I accepted his/her medical decision and treatment.

This release and waiver of any and all claims, known or unknown, arising out of my conversations with Coach on or after this date is complete and without reservation and is binding on myself and any of my heirs or assigns. Furthermore, I agree that a facsimile copy of this signed agreement shall be as binding as the original in every way.

Signed: _____

Print Name: _____

Date: _____